GERONTOLOGICAL PHARMACOLOGY

A RESOURCE
FOR
HEALTH
PRACTITIONERS

GERONTOLOGICAL PHARMACOLOGY

A RESOURCE FOR HEALTH PRACTITIONERS

JOAN E. OPPENEER, R.N., M.S.N.

Professor Emerita,
University of Wisconsin-Milwaukee
School of Nursing; Consultant, Gerontological
Nursing, Milwaukee, Wisconsin

THORA M. VERVOREN, R.Ph., B.S.

Director, Pharmacy Service,
Columbia Hospital, Milwaukee, Wisconsin

The C. V. Mosby Company

ST. LOUIS • TORONTO • LONDON   1983

MOSBY

A TRADITION OF PUBLISHING EXCELLENCE

Editor: Julie Cardamon
Assistant editor: Bess Arends
Manuscript editor: John Middleton
Book design: Jeanne Bush
Cover design: Diane Beasley
Production: Carol O'Leary, Barbara Merritt

The C.V. Mosby Company
11830 Westline Industrial Drive, St. Louis, Missouri 63141

Library of Congress Cataloging in Publication Data

Oppeneer, Joan E.
  Gerontological pharmacology.

  Bibliography: p.
  Includes index.
  1. Geriatric pharmacology. I. Vervoren, Thora M.
II. Title. [DNLM: 1. Drug therapy—In old age.
WT 100 062g]
RC953.7.O66   1983   615.58′0880565   82-14423
ISBN 0-8016-3739-2

AC/VH/VH 9 8 7 6 5 4 3 2 1   01/A/086

PREFACE

Eleven percent of the nation's population is over 65 years of age, and this group uses over 25% of the prescribed drugs plus an untold number of over-the-counter medications. The amount and variety of drugs make the older person vulnerable to problems of misuse, significant interactions, and toxicity. We believe that if practitioners were knowledgeable about the aging process and drug therapy, the incidence of drug-related problems would decrease.

The purpose of this book is to provide a resource on drugs taken by older persons. To facilitate an understanding of aspects of the aging process that relate to drug therapy, the content of Chapters 1 through 7 was designed to improve the practitioner's basic knowledge in gerontology. Included in this section are current trends in gerontology, age-related physical changes, pharmacokinetics, drug interactions, misuse and abuse of medications, promoting good nutrition, and teaching the older adult. Aspects of drug therapy are a component of each chapter. Chapters 8 through 16 focus on selected health problems that are amenable to drug therapy. This section is organized according to body systems, with a brief discussion of health problems and commonly used drugs. Information about drugs includes action, dosage, and proper use and precautions. Because of the current emphasis on generic prescribing and the multiplicity of trade names, generic names are used throughout the text. Drug dosages described are within the standard adult ranges, and when documentation was available, specific geriatric dosages were included. The practitioner or student will find that the organization of Chapters 8 through 16 will make the book a useful tool in direct counseling of patients about drugs.

The book was designed for students and practitioners in nursing, pharmacy, and other health professions. As the older population increases, practitioners will continue to function in the traditional settings, hospitals and nursing homes, but there will be an increasing need for such services in community settings and wherever older people gather. This book will be a valuable resource for professionals in helping older persons maintain optimum levels of health. This goal presents the challenge for the future.

We wish to recognize the contributions of Mary Sinclair Rice, Pharm. D., in the review of the manuscript. We also wish to acknowledge the support and assistance of Paula Meyer and Cheryl Kramer who typed the manuscript.

Joan E. Oppeneer
Thora M. Vervoren

CONTENTS

CURRENT TRENDS IN GERONTOLOGY

The dramatic current and projected growth of the older population has stimulated the various health professions to increase their attention to the aging process and the aging population. An examination of population trends is essential as health-care professionals consider the need for specialized knowledge in aging.

DEMOGRAPHICS

Never before have there been so many old people, either numerically or proportionately, nor have they lived to be so old. In the early 1900s life expectancy was 47 years, and today it is 75 years. During that same period, only 4% of the total population was over 65, and today the aged make up 11% of the total population. In the span of 80 years, the number of aged persons moved from one in twenty-five to one in every nine Americans. Population projections indicate an expected growth to 12% of the population by the year 2000 and to 18% by the year 2030.

The newest phenomenon of aging is the graying of the group itself. The proportion of the 75-year and older group is steadily increasing, growing to 38% in 1980. By the year 2000, the proportionate size of this group is expected to reach 44%.

Another significant change in population statistics is the growth of the 85-year and older group, which has increased to approximately 2 million and produced a 47% increase in 7 years. This rate of growth will continue to increase in the next decades. The old-old group, or persons over 85, is especially vulnerable to physical, emotional, and social problems.

More people are reaching old age because of advances in medicine, public health measures, increased health awareness, and improved living conditions. These advances have contributed to the elimination of the disastrous effects of childbirth and childhood diseases and infectious diseases such as cholera, smallpox, and diphtheria. Interestingly, these problems have been fairly well controlled, but with the increasing incidence of chronic illnesses, overall life expectancy has not increased as much as one would expect. Since 1900, life expectancy at birth has increased 25 years and many more people reach age 65, but once there, they can only expect to live about 4 years longer. If illnesses such as cancer and heart disease, which are today's major killers, were eradicated, life expectancy would be further increased. The great increase in the number of aged Americans has a significant effect on the health professions because this growing group will put greater stress on our health-care system as additional services are required.

Sex, marital status, and living arrangements

Women have consistently lived longer than men, which means that there is a discrepancy between the number of men and women that widens with age. At age 65, there are 13 women to every 10 men, and at age 85, 22.4 women for every 10 men. This discrepancy reflects an 8-year difference in the life expectancy of men and women. Women can expect to live 77 years, whereas men can expect to live to age 69. As a result of this age difference, most older men are married (77%), and most older women are widows (52%). This difference increases with age, so 70% of women over 70 are widows (*Facts About Our Older Americans*, 1978).

Marital status contributes to the type of living arrangement chosen by older persons. Of noninstitutionalized men over 65 in 1975, 79% were married and living with family members. Only 17% were living alone or with nonrelatives. By contrast, only 39% of the women of the group were married, and 41% were living alone or with nonrelatives (Somers, 1980). Only 5% of the aged live in institutions, although this number increases to 20% for the over-85 group. However, 20% of all old people can expect to live in a nursing home at some time, and the probability increases to over 50% for persons over 85.

Because of the higher concentration of older persons in the sun belt states, a common misconception exists that most move to this area. Most older persons continue to live in the neighborhoods where they lived during their middle years. They are not a mobile group, and this stability may be economically mandated. A concentration of persons exists in the older homes in the central city as well as in the rural areas. Older persons living in the suburbs can expect more problems with transportation and provision of health services than their peers living in the cities.

Economics

Poverty, not only low income, is a fact of life for millions of the older population. In 1979, 15% of the over-65 group were poor according to the official definition ($4364 for the household of an older couple or $3472 for an older person living alone). Women and minority elderly are heavily represented in this group. About 35% of elderly blacks and 28% of elderly Hispanic persons were poor.

Inadequate income in later years is a major problem confronting older people. The income of persons over 65 is less than half that of groups under 65. This insufficient income places great stress on older persons, whose expenses for medications and health services increase. Problems of noncompliance, malnutrition, and generally poor health care may be partially attributed to low financial status.

Educational status

The level of education achieved by this group is significant to health-care workers who are providing health information. The years of formal education are less, with 4% of the 65 and older group having received no formal education, and 54% having completed the eighth grade. Approximately 84% of blacks in this group have less than a high school education. A broad gap in communication may exist between the older person and the health professional. Health-care providers need to carefully assess the abilities of older persons because some of them are educated to a sophisticated level, whereas others may be unable to read.

Health status

Aging does not cause specific diseases, but certain chronic illnesses are more prevalent among older adults. Hypertension, heart conditions, neuromuscular disorders, mental conditions, digestive conditions, circulatory problems, diabetes, and ear and eye conditions are among the major health problems of older persons. Conversely, acute illnesses are less common among this group. Chronic and degenerative diseases are the major diagnoses and the primary causes of death. Diseases of the heart, malignant neoplasm, and cerebrovascular disease are the leading causes of death. Chronic illness becomes more prevalent, with 80% of persons over 65 reporting one or more illnesses. The presence of multiple pathological conditions and the manifestation of symptoms that are different from younger persons increase the problems of diagnosis and management.

Despite the frequency of chronic illness, only 46% of this group have activity limitations because of the illness, and 40% are limited in major activities (Brody, 1980). The slow onset of many of the illnesses has permitted the older person to adapt successfully to body changes and maintain self-care in daily activities. Vulnerability to illness increases with age, resulting in decreased ability to function and increased need for services. Shanas (1979) estimates that about one fourth of the elderly residing in the community require home-care services, which includes the 15% who are bedfast, home-bound, or cannot go out without difficulty.

With an increased focus on health awareness, the older adult group also has participated in self-assessment. Despite the high percentage of chronic illness, most elderly view themselves as healthy when compared with others their own age. Self-health assessment may be more significant than the professional evaluation of medical status in predicting general emotional state and behavior. Approximately two thirds of this group rated their health as excellent or good, whereas poor health was reported by 9% of the population studied. The statistics from health assessment as well as functional assessment indicate that the elderly are not frail and sick but that wide variability exists within the group.

IMPACT ON THE HEALTH-CARE SYSTEM

The elderly population makes up 11% of the U.S. population but uses more than 27% of the health-care dollar, a percentage that continues to rise (Lamy, 1980). The use of services is reflected in utilization of institutional facilities, with approximately 30% of the persons in general medical-surgical units over age 65. Most persons in nursing homes are also over age 65. In 1975, 18% of the older population was hospitalized. As age increases, the rate of hospitalization and the average length of stay per patient increase. Older people, regardless of the type of illness or injury, tend to be confined to bed and restricted in activity longer than younger persons do. The period of recovery is longer because the aged body responds more slowly to the stresses of illness.

The increased number of older persons in nursing homes is also significant. Persons up to the age of 64 spend minimum time living in nursing homes, but that number progressively increases, with persons 65 to 74 requiring 4.4 days per year, persons 75 to 84 requiring 21 days per year, and persons over 85 requiring 86.4 days per year (Lamy, 1980). Factors increasing the need for institutionalization are living alone, never having been married or being separated, having few or no children, and being female.

Older persons visit physicians only slightly more often than younger people do, despite the greater frequency of chronic illness and impairment. The elderly accounted for 13% of all physician visits in 1975. The average number of visits that year for all ages was 5.1; persons 65 and over averaged 6.6 visits. The percentage of persons visiting a physician during a given year was similar for all age groups (Yurik, 1980). Most physician visits occur in offices, but with the rising cost of health care, many persons receive care in outpatient clinics. Patients are beginning to seek alternative forms of health care from newly emerging groups of health-care professionals. Geriatric nurse practitioners certified by the American Nurses' Association provide primary care to older persons. Unfortunately, many persons do not seek care because of economic reasons, lack of qualified practitioners, and general discontent with the health-care system. The infrequency of health-care visits may be partially responsible for noncompliance and other drug problems that commonly occur in this population.

As the percentage of older persons with chronic illness increases, so will the use of drugs, placing an added burden on the financial status of the individual and society. Chronic illness requires the use of drugs, not for cure but to control symptoms or to control progression of the disease. Consequently, older persons receive 25% of all prescription drugs. In the early 1970s, older persons received an average of 13 to 14 prescription drugs per year, and in 1979 that number had increased to 17.9 (Butler, 1981). The cost of drugs can be staggering for persons with fixed incomes for whom chronic illness extends over a number of years. For example, the approximate annual cost for the arthritic patient taking ibuprofen is $400; for the hypertensive patient taking propranolol, $275; and for the depressed patient taking amitriptyline, $200. It has been estimated that 20% of the older person's out-of-pocket expenditures are for medicines.

Impact on the health professions

The health professions are responding to the growing older population through the institution of courses that increase the professional's expertise in working with older patients. Selection of practice sites in clinics, nursing homes, gerontology-geriatric centers, and the more traditional hospital settings provides opportunities to use this expertise in direct patient contact. Continuing education courses for health practitioners in the areas of aging are beginning to fulfill the need for persons already in professional practice. These offerings for students and practitioners must expand and be made more available if the elderly are to be better served. Predictions indicate that current graduates of professional programs may find that by the year 2000, 60% to 70% of patients will be elderly.

If more of the older persons are to be cared for in their homes, practitioners will need to be aware of the multiple health problems that can occur. The detection of alterations in health, through skillful observations of signs and symptoms and responses to medications, is the responsibility of nurses, pharmacists, and other professionals. These same people may become involved in community primary prevention services that are designed to prevent disease from occurring through good health-care practices. Reimbursement for health promotion services by government and private agencies will provide an incentive for development and continued expansion.

Having an understanding of who old people are, where they live, what their characteristics are, and what their health status is provides background information that gives insight into the needs of older persons. This is only the beginning. To better understand and meet these needs, especially as they relate to pharmacology, the practitioner must understand the changes that take place in the aging body, the pharmacokinetics of aging, common health problems and related drug management, strategies for teaching individuals and groups about medications, and problems of drug abuse.

Health practitioners share a common core of knowledge, and part of this core should be in the area of gerontology, the study of the aging process. Beyond the common core, each professional brings expertise that must be shared with well and ill older persons and with other professionals.

If health-care professionals are to be influential in providing the care older people deserve, they must expand their knowledge, become involved in research efforts, be aware of national health policy that affects older persons and the professions, and generally become advocates for the aged.

REFERENCES

Brody, S.J.: The graying of America, Hospitals **54:**63, 1980.
Butler, R.N.: Pharmacy's contribution to geriatric care, Drug Intell. Clin. Pharm. **15:**569, 1981.
Lamy, P.: Prescribing for the elderly, Littleton, Mass., 1980, John Wright-PSG, Inc.
Shanas, E.: Social myth as hypothesis, Gerontologist **19:**13, 1979.
Somers, A.: Demographics can help guide social policy, Hospitals **54:**67, 1980.
U.S. Department of Health, Education, and Welfare: Facts about our older Americans, Pub. No. (OHDS) 79-20006, Washington, D.C., 1978, U.S. Government Printing Office.
Yurik, A., and others: The aged person and the nursing process, New York, 1980, Appleton-Century-Crofts.

SUGGESTED READINGS

Atchley, R.: The social forces in later life, ed. 3, Belmont, Calif., 1980, Wadsworth Publishing Co.
Butler, R., and Lewis, M.: Aging and mental health: positive psychological approaches, ed. 2, St. Louis, 1979, The C.V. Mosby Co.
Hendricks, J., and Hendricks, C.: Aging in mass society, Cambridge, Mass., 1977, Winthrop Publishers, Inc.
Rossman, I., editor: Clinical geriatrics, ed. 2, Philadelphia, 1979, J.B. Lippincott Co.

AGE-RELATED PHYSICAL CHANGES

2

Because of the interrelatedness of all body systems, the process of aging has a distinct effect on each system. Having the knowledge of these various changes that usually occur with aging, the health professional can more readily anticipate the action drugs may produce on the aging body. The practitioner can also discuss with the patient those changes that are age related and suggest medical referral for those that appear to be due to pathological conditions.

Age-related changes begin at birth and continue throughout life. These changes that occur in body tissues differ in nature and time of occurrence. Alterations, which are very individualized to each person, may be so gradual that the person adapts to them, and unless some stress is placed on the body or body system the person may be unaware of the change.

Goldman (1979) has identified four characteristics of aging as (1) universal, (2) progressive, (3) decremental, and (4) intrinsic. The universality of aging removes it from consideration as a merely pathological condition and identifies it as a natural phenomenon. Because of the simultaneous occurrence of multiple pathological conditions with aging, differentiation of normal aging becomes a difficult process. Longitudinal studies extending from middle to old age will continue to verify normal aging changes. The progressive and decremental characteristics decrease the ability of the person to interact with the environment and relate to the increasing risk of approaching death. Most of the aging changes are intrinsic and will occur in a definable pattern, but extrinsic factors are also responsible for a host of changes and may hasten those related to age.

This chapter presents the identified normal age changes of each body system in the older adult. The information will be useful in planning intervention strategies, providing health education programs to individuals and groups, and discussing patients with other groups of health professionals.

Specific suggestions for intervention strategies are included with each system.

GENERAL APPEARANCE

The body tissue that undergoes the greatest change throughout life is fat (Rossman, 1979). The subcutaneous fat that fills out and rounds the body shows a general decrease in older age. As a result, contours become more sharp, hollows more apparent, and bony landmarks more prominent. Peripheral body parts also evidence these changes. Legs and arms appear thin in relation to the abdomen. Tendons, bones, and vessels of the feet and hands become more apparent when the fatty layer diminishes. The fatty layer around the eye orbit disappears, giving the eyes a deep or sunken appearance. Formerly firm breast tissue begins to atrophy with the resultant sagging, pendulous breasts characteristic of older women.

General changes in body composition that show a decrease include plasma volume, total body water, and extracellular fluid. Surprisingly, total body fat increases, but total body weight decreases, which is due primarily to a decrease in lean body mass.

Recommendations for intervention

Since subcutaneous fat helps to insulate the body, its loss causes the older person to chill more readily. This change, coupled with the generally lowered ability in thermoregulation, may make the adjustment to cool temperatures more difficult and possibly hazardous. Attention must be given to requests for warm clothing, extra blankets, and warmer room temperature. Older persons who go outdoors in cold weather must be protected from chilling. More vulnerable persons in this group are those whose activity is restricted by disability and the effects of drugs such as central nervous system (CNS) depressants.

INTEGUMENTARY SYSTEM

Changes in the skin, hair, and nails are the most evident alterations in the aging body.

Skin

Wrinkled skin, particularly of the face and neck and exposed body parts, may be one of the first signs of aging. Factors influencing the onset of these wrinkles are skin elasticity, maintenance of subcutaneous fat, exposure to the sun and heat, and the general state of nutrition and health. The epithelial layer of the skin thins, and collagen becomes more rigid. Loss of body fat intensifies the wrinkling, and the skin becomes more lax because of loss of elasticity.

The gravitational pull is responsible for changes that affect the eyelids, ears, jowls, and general facial expression. Skin color may change to a uniformly pale tone, which is affected by changes in the capillaries. Areas of the body exposed to extensive sun radiation may become yellowish and leathery. The brown pigmented spots appearing on the hands, wrists, and sometimes the face are known as senile lentigo. These harmless areas are commonly known as liver spots but have no relationship to the liver.

Nails

Nail growth decreases with age, and the nails become hard, thick, and brittle. The latter changes are probably related to changes in peripheral circulation and are complicated by the presence of fungal infections of the nail beds.

Hair

Hair, which undergoes changes in color, texture, and distribution, is affected by genetic, endocrine, and age factors. A change in hair color to gray, beginning at the temples, is caused by decreasing amounts of melanin in the hair itself. In both sexes, facial hair tends to increase, while hair on other parts of the body decreases and may eventually disappear. Balding occurs in varying amounts in both men and women and follows a characteristic pattern with loss at the vertex and frontal areas. The pattern of balding is sex linked, with the mother passing the trait on to her sons.

The loss of pubic and axillary hair in women is probably related to hormonal changes and begins in the postmenopausal period. The fine hair on the ears of young men changes to coarse, longer hairs located primarily on their ear lobes as they become old men.

Recommendations for intervention

Prevention has a definite role in the degree of skin change that occurs. Protection from the sun's rays, maintenance of body weight, good nutrition, and exercise, particularly of the facial muscles, do have a positive effect. Informing the younger patient of these measures of prevention and helping the aging patient regarding expected changes in the integumentary system are clearly professional responsibilities. The older person should be made aware of the need for fewer baths, the use of emollients after the bath, and drying the skin by blotting with an absorbent towel. Inexpensive lotions and creams will prevent some of the extreme dryness and flaking that may occur. However, even expensive creams and lotions will not prevent the eventual skin changes.

Caring for hard, rigid toenails may be problematic for older persons who have visual and musculoskeletal changes. The elderly diabetic patient is especially vulnerable to nail and foot problems. When the nails are soft following a bath, they should be cut straight across. The assistance of another person or the services of a podiatrist may be recommended. Recommendations for foot care are included in a later chapter in this book.

MUSCULOSKELETAL SYSTEM

The more apparent changes in the musculoskeletal system that affect the person's functional ability include loss of muscle strength, flexibility, equilibrium, and speed of motion.

Height and posture

A progressive decline in height, particularly in the trunk, becomes evident in persons of both sexes as they become older. In the middle years as the spongy intervertebral disks begin to shrink, a decrease in stature becomes evident. In the later years, especially in women, the vertebrae begin to narrow, and the characteristic appearance of a shorter trunk with long arms and legs occurs. The narrowing of the vertebrae is caused by fracture and collapse associated with osteoporosis. Kyphosis combined with loss of height is compensated for by a backward tilting of the head, which further reduces the occiput-to-shoulder distance. Another postural change contributing to changes in height is slight flexion of the knees and hips. These alterations in height and posture have a distinct effect on the person's mobility and equilibrium. In addition, changes in posture affect the functioning of body organs.

Muscles

Atrophy of muscle fibers that are replaced by fat results in decreased strength, flexibility, and endurance. Changes in muscle strength are particularly prominent in the arms, legs, and back, with back pain a common complaint.

Bones

The bones, deprived of adequate absorption of calcium and affected by the lack of the necessary stress achieved by exercise, become porous and brittle. Osteoporosis may occur and increases the incidence of fractures, particularly among women, and is a major cause of morbidity and mortality in the aged.

Recommendations for intervention

Because persons who exercise regularly do not lose as much bone or muscle mass, a regular program of exercise for all persons is recommended. Group exercise programs led by a capable health professional have proven to be effective. The concern for general mobility and possible loss of equilibrium may necessitate the use of a cane, chair, walker, or other means of support when walking or exercising. Changes in lean body mass that may affect the distribution of drugs necessitates careful observation.

NERVOUS SYSTEM

The aging process affects the structure and function of the CNS, but the reserve capacity of the cells permits the brain to function adequately when the person is not exposed to stressful conditions. Clinical manifestations are seldom exhibited except when the person is exposed to stress, electrolyte imbalance, poor nutrition, depressant drugs, and disruptive experiences.

Neuronal changes

Because neurons are postmitotic, they are not replaced when lost. The rate of loss differs for different parts of the brain. Fortunately, humans have a very large number of cells, far more than will ever be used in a lifetime. Since brain cells decrease by about 1% per year after the age of 50, a person of 70 may have lost 20% of them. The loss of thousands of cells daily does not necessarily affect functioning or impair behavior. The cells that remain also undergo some changes that may compromise functioning. Lipofuscin, a brownish pigment in nerve and other body cells, accumulates in the nerve cells, and the quantity correlates with age. However, it is not known if it has any effect on cell function.

Brain circulation

Age-related changes that occur in cerebral blood flow and use of oxygen have been well studied. Goldman (1979) reports that the following progression of values occurs between ages 17 and 80: (1) mean arterial pressure remains constant, (2) cerebral blood flow declines, (3) cerebral oxygen consumption rate declines, and (4) cerebrovascular resistance increases. There is a significant decrease in cerebral blood flow and metabolism that occurs with the aging process, and this decrease has an effect on total body functioning.

Nerve conduction

Nerve conduction velocity decreases after the age of 50, with estimates of decline ranging from 10% to 15% by the eighth decade. The change, which is reported to be greater in women than men, is probably caused by a decrease in individual cell functioning. The general slowing of reflexes that occurs is partially the result of this nerve conduction decline.

Recommendations for intervention

The reserve capacity of the brain to function and control body functioning remains fairly constant throughout life. A sudden change in function should be investigated through a health history taken by the health professional. The stress of physical or emotional illness, the ingestion of prescribed or over-the-counter (OTC) drugs, or malnutrition may be responsible for change in function.

To decrease the incidence of dizziness and fainting caused by decreased cerebral circulation, the patient should be advised to move slowly from a recumbent to an upright position and to avoid positions of extreme neck flexion or hyperextension.

The change in nerve transmission velocity can be accommodated by allowing the person a longer time to respond to a stimulus and by advising that this change can occur with aging.

SENSORY SYSTEM

The entire sensory system undergoes progressive changes that affect functioning and the enjoyment of life through seeing, hearing, smelling, touching, and tasting. Visual and auditory changes are discussed in Chapter 7.

Sense of touch

A general loss of sensitivity to touch occurs in the older adult, but the loss is highly variable. Some changes may be pathologically based and caused by old injuries or circulatory abnormalities. The skin on the palm of the hand

and sole of the foot has a decreased sensitivity that does not occur in the hair-covered body surfaces.

The older adult also undergoes changes that impair the ability to cope with alterations in environmental temperatures. Current studies in hypothermia reveal multiple problems that may be present in older persons, including the ability to adapt to cold, that increase the danger of hypothermia.

The older person also has change in pain sensitivity, which may be due to degenerative changes in the peripheral nervous system and receptors. Pain may not be felt when a pathological condition exists, and sites of pain may not follow familiar patterns.

Recommendations for intervention

A decrease in the sense of touch affects the person's ability to localize the source of a stimulus, such as the heat from a burner on a stove. As a result, injury may occur. Coupled with the changes in the sensitivity to pain, the person may be unaware of the pressure caused by a tight-fitting shoe until tissue trauma has occurred. Advice needs to be given about the hazards of hypothermia and methods of prevention achieved by warm clothing and comfortable room temperatures. Safety is the major theme in prevention of problems associated with changes in tactile sensation.

Sense of taste

With aging, there is a decrease in the sense of taste, which is probably caused by a decrease in the number of taste buds. Estimates indicate that the average person loses over half the taste buds by age 75. Other changes affecting the sense of taste include a history of pipe smoking, decreased saliva, and cellular changes of the oral cavity. Elderly persons report an increased sensitivity to bitterness and decreased sensitivity to sweetness and saltiness. This may be caused by the loss of taste buds that are sensitive to salty and sweet stimulation and are located at the tip and base of the tongue. The change in sensitivity may also be explained by the higher threshold of the remaining taste buds, which require greater stimulation to give the person a sense of satisfaction.

Recommendations for intervention

Because changes in the sense of taste can affect a person's appetite, more highly seasoned food may be preferred. Frequently there are food restrictions imposed by excess weight or altered cardiovascular status, so the use of herbs, lemon juice, and other seasonings are suggested to enhance the flavor of food and decrease the need for salt. The sensitivity to sour and bitter flavors should be noted when recommending flavor enhancers and when suggesting methods of taking medications. In situations in which medications may be sour or bitter, an alternative form may be recommended if available.

Sense of smell

The sense of smell declines minimally with aging. This alteration may be caused by a decline in the number of fibers in the olfactory nerve. Because healthy persons show little decline, it is speculated that the alteration may be caused by ill health and extrinsic factors such as occupational odors and toxic agents.

Recommendations for intervention

A decrease in the sense of smell eliminates warnings of the dangers of smoke, gas, and toxic odors that may be present in the environment. The use of fire alarms, electric instead of gas stoves, or safety caps for gas stove jets is advisable. The person may also be unaware of unpleasant personal and household odors and should be advised if they are present. Because the senses of smell and taste are so closely related, suggestions offered previously to improve food flavors are recommended.

RESPIRATORY SYSTEM

The identification of age-related changes in the respiratory system is complicated by the environmental effects of air pollution, exposure to occupational hazards, and the results of smoking throughout one's life or living with one who smokes. When there are no known pathological conditions, older persons are capable of adapting to the changes. However, with exercise or stress, dyspnea and other symptoms of distress may occur.

Skeletal changes affecting lung capacity occur with age. The following changes can decrease the compliance of the chest wall: (1) increase of the anteroposterior diameter of the chest, (2) kyphosis, (3) osteoporosis, (4) vertebral collapse, (5) calcification of rib cartilages, and (6) reduced rib mobility. Changes in the muscles affect the ability of the thoracic cavity to increase and decrease in size.

The lungs become more rigid with age, and this rigidity reduces the vital capacity, or the amount of air that can be expelled from the lungs after full expiration. The residual volume, or air left in the lungs, shows a linear increase with aging. The number of alveoli decreases, and the size of those remaining also shows a decrease. Thickness of the alveoli and capillary membranes, combined with other respiratory changes, decreases the availability of oxygen.

Recommendations for intervention

Changes in the respiratory system decrease the ability of the older person to cough forcefully enough to expel secretions that may accumulate and possibly cause an infection. To prevent this problem and other potential respiratory problems, the following measures are recommended: (1) a regular program of physical activity to promote muscle tone and general fitness, (2) good posture, (3) coughing and deep breathing exercises, (4) avoidance of persons with respiratory infections, (5) avoiding smoking and smoke-filled rooms, and (6) drinking sufficient fluids to liquify secretions if a respiratory infection should occur.

CARDIOVASCULAR SYSTEM

The cardiovascular system, which is composed of the heart and blood vessels, undergoes changes that can generally be accommodated unless the person is subjected to physical or emotional stress.

Heart

The aging heart continues to function adequately under ordinary circumstances but, as other body systems also do, loses much of its functional reserve. Contrary to popular opinion, the heart size does not increase with age, but a change in size suggests a pathological condition. The amount of fatty tissue and pigment may increase, and the valves become more thickened and rigid. The most significant age-related change is the alteration in cardiac output, which is reduced by 30% to 40% between the ages of 25 and 65 (Goldman, 1979). This change has a marked effect on the elimination of drugs by the liver and kidneys. Stroke volume is decreased. Maximum oxygen consumption declines with age as the rate of cardiac output decreases. The resting heart rate remains essentially the same throughout life, but the length of time to return to basal levels is lengthened following exercise.

Blood vessels

The vascular system, especially the arteries, shows greater evidence of changes than the heart does. Elasticity of the vessels is affected by progressive fraying, splitting, and fragmenting of the elastic fibers. Some of the calcium lost by the bones is deposited in the blood vessels. Simultaneously, the collagen in the vessels increases, and the cross-linking of this material further compromises elasticity. The reduced cardiac output and vessel changes affect blood flow to various body organs, but the change is not equal to all parts. Flow to the brain and coronary artery vessels decreases only minimally, but flow to the kidneys and liver is significantly reduced.

Peripheral resistance causes the heart to pump harder, and as a result, systolic and diastolic blood pressure may increase. Caird and Judge (1974) indicate that older persons without cardiac problems and hypertension disorders do have higher blood pressure. Opinions vary about the normal range of blood pressure in older persons, but current therapy indicates the need to control elevations conservatively.

Recommendations for intervention

Current beliefs about the effects of life-style on the incidence of cardiovascular problems, including hypertension, indicate the need for preventive health measures throughout one's life. A program of regular exercise, weight control, well-balanced diet, relief of stress, and avoidance of smoking are also important for older persons, although the exercise program may need to be altered.

In situations in which the aging heart and vessels limit activity, a very moderate but regular program is recommended. Also, pacing activities will allow the person to accomplish them without placing added strain on the cardiovascular system.

Older persons should also have their blood pressure monitored at health centers, professional offices, or other reputable agencies offering this service. A system of referral for medical follow-up should be part of any monitoring service.

Postural hypotension is fairly common in older persons and may be caused or exaggerated by medications. The discussion of safety measures, such as slowly rising from a lying to a sitting position and maintaining a sitting position for several minutes before standing, is important as a precautionary measure.

GASTROINTESTINAL SYSTEM

Multiple changes affect the gastrointestinal tract, but generally the older adult accommodates to the change and functions adequately.

Oral changes

The oral cavity undergoes a series of changes that have an effect on chewing and ultimately on the digestion of food. Approximately half of the population over 65 years old have lost their teeth, primarily as a consequence of poor dental hygiene, periodontal disease, and general neglect. Lack of teeth and ill-fitting dentures contribute to improperly masticated food, which ultimately affects digestion.

Taste buds and oral mucosa undergo changes, and the salivary flow decreases and thickens. Dry mouth is a common complaint and may also be related to taking medications such as anticholinergics and tranquilizers. Absorption of buccal medications may be delayed because of the lack of salivary flow.

Esophagus

The esophagus undergoes changes in peristalsis, which can be complicated by poorly masticated food. The peristaltic movements are decreased, the esophagus is emptied more slowly, and there is a delay in emptying that can result in a dilatation of the lower esophagus.

Stomach

Gastric motility is decreased, accompanied by a generally lessened tone, which results in delayed emptying. These changes result in a generally slowed down process. Absorption, which can be affected by the motility, condition of the absorptive surface, and blood flow to the gastric area, has an effect on absorption of vitamins and minerals. Vitamins B_1 and B_{12}, iron, and calcium may be absorbed less efficiently because of the decrease in acid and enzymes.

Liver and gallbladder

The function of the liver and gallbladder is generally maintained despite the changes they undergo. Some inefficiency may be manifested by alterations in fat absorption, lower tolerance to fat, and accumulation of medications that are detoxified primarily by the liver.

Colon

Much attention has been given to the constipation problems of older persons. Physiological changes responsible for some of these problems include decreased muscle tone which in turn affects peristalsis, decreased tone of the internal sphincter, and decreased tone of the anal sphincter. The aging changes combined with a diet low in roughage, inadequately masticated food, insufficient fluid intake, and lack of exercise also contribute to the development of constipation. Changes in general bowel tissue elasticity and lack of dietary fiber are responsible for the overuse of laxatives and the incidence of diverticuli common in older adults.

Recommendations for intervention

Although the gastrointestinal tract undergoes changes, it essentially accommodates to the change and permits the older person to function without problems. Areas of teaching to promote better functioning include (1) good oral hygiene and dental referral as needed, (2) the importance of nutritious, tasty meals eaten at regular times, (3) sources of essential vitamins, (4) adequate fluid intake, and (5) a regular program of exercise. In situations in which a dry mouth persists, the use of ice chips, mouthwash, chewing gum, and sugarless hard candy is recommended. A regular program of oral hygiene that includes using a soft brush to massage the gums and tongue also helps to control the problems of a dry mouth.

URINARY SYSTEM

The kidneys are capable of functioning adequately despite the decrease in cells, which is primarily due to nephron loss. The kidney changes suggest that (1) filtration rate is decreased, (2) excretory and reabsorptive functions of the renal tubules are decreased, and (3) acid-base balance is more easily disrupted when a person is exposed to stress. Arteriosclerosis and other vessel changes affect renal blood flow.

The remaining urinary structures, ureters, bladder, and urethra, begin to lose tone with the aging process. The bladder is particularly affected, because with the decrease in tone, the person is unable to completely empty the bladder, and the residual urine increases the risk of infections. The bladder capacity decreases by approximately half its normal volume, resulting in more frequent and more urgent urination. The warning period may decrease, resulting in urinary incontinence.

Recommendations for intervention

Older persons may be hesitant to discuss problems related to urinary changes because of feeling sensitive about the subject. They may begin to withdraw socially because of the embarrassment of incontinence. Nocturia also becomes a problem. Suggestions that can be made to the older person include (1) provision of ready access to toilet facilities, (2) regular emptying of the bladder, (3) bladder training exercises, (4) pelvic floor exercises, (5) use of absorbent disposable pads as a precautionary measure, and (6) adequate fluid intake as a means of decreasing the risk of bladder infections. If nocturia is present, sufficient night lighting is essential as a safety measure in the prevention of falls.

ENDOCRINE SYSTEM

Multiple age-related changes occur in the endocrine system, but this section will be limited to alterations of the pancreas, thyroid gland, and gonads.

Pancreas

Older persons have a decline in the ability to metabolize glucose. This impairment may occur as a result of a decrease in the amount of insulin secreted by the pancreas or reduced peripheral sensitivity to circulating insulin. Increased levels of blood glucose in older adults must be carefully evaluated before treatment is instituted. Various medications, such as thiazide diuretics and glucocorticoids, may affect blood glucose control.

Thyroid gland

A decrease in thyroid activity is evidenced by slowing of the metabolic rate and use of oxygen. However, hypothyroidism seldom occurs because of the reserve capacity of the gland.

Gonads

Ovarian estrogen is no longer produced by the ovaries following menopause. Estrogen in males, produced by the adrenal glands, shows very minimum age-related change. Progesterone produced by the ovaries and placenta, and to a lesser extent by the testes and adrenal cortex, declines significantly following the reproductive period. Blood levels of testosterone reportedly decrease.

Specific changes that occur in the female reproductive system include (1) thinning of the vaginal mucosa, (2) decrease in size of the vagina, with less elasticity, (3) decrease in vaginal secretions, which also become less acidic, and (4) decrease in the size of the uterus and ovaries. Changes occurring in the male reproductive system are as follows: (1) testes decrease in size and become more firm, (2) fewer sperm are produced, and (3) the incidence of prostatic hypertrophy increases and is further aggravated by anticholinergic drugs. Despite the changes that occur in men and women, the desire for sexual activity continues. Intercourse may become less frequent and may take longer to accomplish, but the partners continue to find satisfaction in the sexual relationship.

Recommendations for intervention

Creating consumer awareness about the changes affecting the endocrine system, particularly those changes that involve the reproductive system, is a responsibility that can be shared by health professionals. Studies regarding sexuality in this population have exploded the myths about lack of ability and desirability. Sexual activity continues to be an interest and concern of older adults.

SUMMARY

This chapter has explored the physiological changes that occur as people grow older. The changes, identified by body systems, are closely interrelated, with changes in one system affecting another. Emphasis must be made that these changes are highly individual; the time at which and degree to which they occur vary from one person to another. A healthy life-style is known to delay the changes.

REFERENCES

Caird, F., and Judge, D.: Assessment of the elderly patient, Marshfield, Mass., 1974, Pitman Publishing, Inc.

Goldman, R.: Decline in organ function with age. In Rossman, I., editor: Clinical geriatrics, Philadelphia, 1979, J.B. Lippincott Co.

Rossman, I.: Anatomy of aging. In Rossman, I., editor: Clinical geriatrics, Philadelphia, 1979, J.B. Lippincott Co.

SUGGESTED READINGS

Carnevali, D., and Patrick, M.: Nursing management for the elderly, Philadelphia, 1979, J.B. Lipincott Co.

Futrel, M., and others: Primary health care for the older adult, Boston, 1980, Duxbury Press.

Libow, L.S., and Sherman, F.J., editors: The core of geriatric medicine: a guide for students and practitioners, St. Louis, 1981, The C.V. Mosby Co.

Riley, G.: How aging affects drug therapy, U.S. Pharmacist **2:**29, 1977.

Saxon, S., and Ehen, M.: Physical change and aging: a guide for the helping professions, New York, 1978, Tiresias Press.

3

PHARMACOKINETICS AND AGING

Pharmacokinetics, the study of the disposition of drugs in the body, deals with rates of absorption, distribution, metabolism, and elimination of drugs. An understanding of the principles governing these processes in the body is necessary before we look at how the response of the aged to drugs is affected.

To conceptualize drug kinetics, the body has been depicted as a system of compartments into which a drug is absorbed and distributed. The one-compartment model is the simplest and most useful in describing the kinetics of drugs that are rapidly distributed throughout the body.

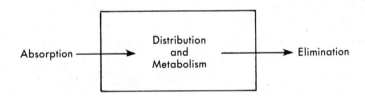

As the complexity of the processes increases, multicompartment systems are projected to represent various organs, tissues, and fluid areas of the body such as plasma and extracellular fluid. An example might be a central compartment into which the drug is absorbed and distributed and a peripheral compartment into which the drug redistributes. The effect of this second compartment is to prolong the length of time the drug remains in the body before it is eliminated.

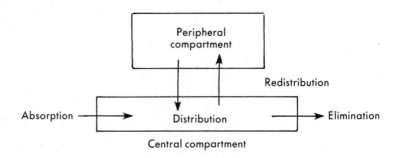

ABSORPTION

To produce systemic effects, drugs must be absorbed into the body. Absorption is controlled by factors such as the route of administration, formulation of the drug product, physicochemical properties of the drug, and internal environment of the patient. The measurement of the rate and extent of absorption of a drug is known as bioavailability. Bioavailability studies are used to determine generic equivalence between the same drug manufactured by more than one source.

To be absorbed, drugs in the form of tablets and capsules must disintegrate and become dissolved in the gastric juices. Ideally, 100% of an administered dose should reach the systemic circulation unchanged after oral absorption. However, this is not the case for many drugs because of the factors listed previously that control absorption. Absorption following intravenous administration is by definition 100% complete. Absolute bioavailability is defined as the fraction of the total dose absorbed intact and is usually determined by comparing the extent of oral with intravenous absorption following administration of equal doses. Measurement of urinary excretion for drugs that are largely excreted unchanged in the urine is another indicator of bioavailability. When two oral products of the same drug are compared, the term "relative bioavailability" is used. This is defined as the fraction of the dose absorbed to the fraction absorbed of an equivalent dose of another oral product. The products are administered at different times but under similar conditions.

Differences in bioavailability between the same drug and dosage form produced by various manufacturers may result in decreased effectiveness or toxic reactions because of the extent of the absorption. Lists of drugs with possible problems of this type have been published by the American Pharmaceutical Association.

Measurement of the concentration of a drug in the blood or plasma, known as "Cp," characterizes the kinetics of that drug. Often the pharmacological effect of the drug is proportional to the Cp. The rate of absorption of a drug can be determined from Cp studies taken at various time intervals. Plotting these data gives a plasma level time curve for a single dose of a drug as illustrated below:

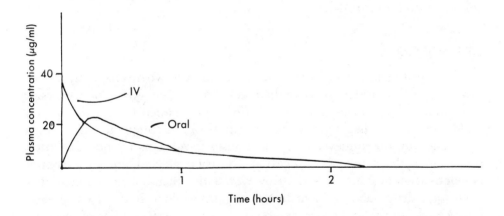

The fraction of the dose absorbed is indicated by the area under the plasma level time curve. For rapid onset of drug action, a rapid peak Cp to produce the therapeutic effect is desirable. To produce a sustained effect, a low peak level indicative of slower absorption may be necessary. Sometimes high peak levels produce toxic effects. With other drugs, steady state plasma levels are produced because of accumulation of the drug following chronic administration.

DISTRIBUTION

Distribution is the process by which drugs are delivered to various sites in the body. Following absorption, drugs may enter a variety of body fluids and tissues according to the chemical characteristics of the drug. The measure of the compartment into which the drug enters is termed the volume of distribution, known as "Vd." Vd is defined as the amount of drug in the body divided by the Cp. The amount of drug in the body, or "Ab," just after a dose is given will be equal to the dose, assuming that the drug is completely absorbed. Therefore the Vd can be calculated from the dose and the estimation of the Cp at the time the dose is given.

$$Vd = \frac{Ab}{Cp}$$

Variation in the Vd is produced by a number of factors including total body water, lean body mass, body fat, sex, renal function, and the extent of drug binding to albumin and other plasma proteins. The portion of a drug bound to plasma protein remains inactive until displaced by other protein-bound drugs. Displacement can result in possible toxicity because of high concentrations of free drug.

METABOLISM

The site of metabolism for most drugs is the liver, where enzymatic action produces metabolic derivatives called metabolites. The process of conversion to metabolites enhances drug elimination and is called biotransformation.

Metabolites are usually more polar, water-soluble compounds that can be eliminated by the kidneys. Types of biotransformations include oxidation, reduction, hydrolysis, and conjugation. The usual effect of biotransformation is inactivation or detoxification. However, active metabolites are generated from some drugs, and in other drugs no pharmacological activity is present until conversion to an active metabolite takes place. Examples of biotransformations from inactive or active drugs to active or more active metabolites include allopurinol to alloxanthine, amitriptyline to nortriptyline, methyldopa to methylnorepinephrine, and propranolol to 4-hydroxypropranolol.

The enzymatic action of the liver may be increased or inhibited by some drugs that may lead to drug toxicity or reduced activity unless dosage adjustments are made. This drug action on liver enzymes is the reason for many drug interactions.

The hepatic metabolism of drugs in disease states is unpredictable because of the diverse effects of different hepatic diseases on the metabolic functions of the liver and variations in the liver blood flow.

Another pharmacokinetic concept is the first-pass effect, which identifies a process of metabolism that occurs between the site of absorption and the systemic circulation. First-pass effect may occur in the gastrointestinal epithelium, mesenteric and portal blood, or the liver following oral or deep rectal administration. The clinical importance of the first-pass effect depends primarily on the rate of absorption, the rate of metabolism, and the metabolic capacity of the enzyme systems for a particular drug and results in variations in the bioavailability of the drug. Low bioavailability of the drug occurs if the metabolic capacity is high and the rate of metabolism is fast following absorption. The first-pass metabolizing system may become saturated with increasing doses, and an increase in bioavailability results.

ELIMINATION

Drugs may be eliminated from the systemic circulation by different pathways, such as urine, bile, saliva, sweat, breast milk, and alveolar air. The major pathways are via the kidney into the urine and via the liver into the feces.

Most drugs are absorbed, distributed, and eliminated by a process known as first-order kinetics. A first-order process means that the rate of drug excretion and the rate of drug transfer between compartments are directly related to the concentration of the drug. For each of these processes there is a unit of time called the half-life ($t_{1/2}$) during which the concentration of the drug will change by 50%. The elimination half-life of a drug is a measure of its rate of elimination from the body and is the half-life used for most clinical applications of kinetics.

An important factor in the elimination rate of weakly acidic and basic drugs is the pH of the urine. At low urinary pH values, weak bases are more highly ionized and less readily reabsorbed and therefore excreted more rapidly. At high urinary pH values the reverse is true.

A reliable indicator of kidney function is creatinine clearance laboratory measurements. The normal range is 105 to 150 ml/min for a standard average adult surface area of 1.73 m².

DOSING REGIMENS AND PLASMA LEVELS

The half-life concept is also useful in determining dosing intervals. One dosing regimen based on the half-life is to administer an initial loading dose followed by a maintenance dose every half-life. Drugs with very short or very long half-lives must be dosed differently, with account taken of the therapeutic index or the margin between therapeutic and toxic plasma levels. If a drug has little dose-related toxicity, large amounts can be given at intervals longer than the half-life. Drugs with long half-lives are usually given once daily.

The accumulation of a drug in the body occurs when maintenance doses of the drug are given at intervals less than the half-life. For example, if aminophylline ($t_{1/2}$ = 6 hours) is given every 6 hours, only one half-life passes between doses. Half of the previous dose remains when each subsequent dose is given, and accumulation occurs. The point at which the amount of drug eliminated during the dosing interval equals the amount administered is known as the steady state ($\bar{C}p$). The $\bar{C}p$ for any drug given at a constant interval occurs according to the number of half-lives that have passed. Usually four half-lives or approximately 94% change in concentration is used as the time required to be near the $\bar{C}p$.

Number of half-lives	% Change in concentration
1	50
2	75
3	87.5
4	93.8
5	96.9
6	98.4
7	99.2

Peak and trough levels appear above and below the $\bar{C}p$ on the plasma level time curve shown below, as a result of intermittent dosing.

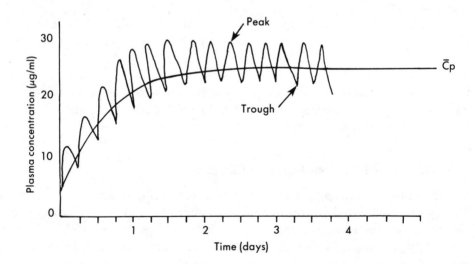

The drug plasma level equates with the patient's clinical response to many drugs, and therefore plasma levels can be helpful in determining dosing regimens in individual patients. Because drug levels are continuously changing, the time to obtain a blood sample for analysis is critical. Trough levels, or levels drawn immediately before the next dose, are valuable for all drugs except those with dosing intervals spanning many half-lives. Peak levels, or levels drawn when the serum concentration is highest, are difficult to anticipate and reproduce. The peak concentration occurs immediately after an intravenous bolus, but the same dose given by any other route attains peak concentration when the rate of absorption no longer exceeds the combined rates of distribution and excretion. In general, a peak level occurs ½ to 2 hours after a nonintravenous dose of a drug under normal absorption processes. Sustained release preparations, parenteral suspensions, and depot injections produce later peaks.

Plasma levels provide useful data about the performance of a drug in a patient. However, accurate assays are not always available, and other patient-related variables often negate or limit their usefulness.

PHARMACOKINETICS AND AGING

Advancing age brings changes in body structure and function as reviewed in Chapter 2. These changes significantly alter the pharmacokinetics—the process governing the absorption, distribution, metabolism, and elimination—of drugs in the elderly population.

Gastrointestinal changes

In general, the ability to absorb both water-soluble and fat-soluble drugs from the upper gastrointestinal tract is unchanged in the older adult. However, absorption is affected by changes in gastrointestinal motility. Drugs such as anticholinergics, tricyclic antidepressants, antihistamines, and phenothiazines slow gastrointestinal motility, allow more time for absorption to occur, and therefore increase drug effects. Drugs such as laxatives increase gastrointestinal motility and may prevent adequate absorption, reducing drug effects. The formation of insoluble and therefore nonabsorbable complexes in the small intestine, such as the insoluble metal complexes formed between tetracycline and calcium and iron salts, reduces absorption.

Changes in absorption may occur because of achlorhydria or hypochlorhydria, in which the decrease in acid production may affect the absorption of weakly acidic drugs such as barbiturates. Other age-related changes that might alter drug absorption include increases in gastric pH and decreases in visceral blood flow. However, few studies of drug absorption have shown that clinically significant changes occur with increasing age.

Changes in body composition

Increasing age-related factors alter the distribution of drugs in the body. Changes in body composition have been noted. The proportion of body fat increases. Total body water, plasma volume, and extracellular fluid decrease. The reduction in lean body mass may affect drug distribution by decreasing the volume in which it can occur and thereby produce higher peak levels. The reduction in total body water may increase the toxicity of water-soluble drugs such as lithium and salicylates in the older adult. Increased fat increases the ability to store fat-soluble compounds such as barbiturates and phenothiazines and increases the risk of toxicity as doses accumulate. Serum albumin concentration decreases with age. Drugs that are highly protein bound, such as propranolol, phenytoin, and indomethacin, have fewer binding sites, and this leads to increased amounts of free drug in the circulation than is calculated from the normal dose. Pharmacological action and toxicity may be increased. Another factor that affects the distribution of drugs is the reduction in cardiac output and the increase in peripheral vascular resistance. Blood flow to the liver and kidney decreases, and more of the cardiac output is distributed to the skeletal muscle, cerebral, and coronary areas.

Changes in liver function

Hepatic metabolism is also affected by the decrease in liver blood flow and the decrease in liver mass. Alterations occur in the $\bar{C}p$ levels of drugs administered intravenously and in the first-pass extraction of orally administered drugs. An age-related reduction in liver microsomal enzymatic activity and inducibility has been found that may lead to reduced drug metabolism, drug accumulation, and toxicity. Drugs that have been demonstrated to have a decreased hepatic metabolism in older adults include diazepam and theophylline. In general, hepatic function is adequate to meet the metabolic demands of the older adult. The effects of aging on the metabolism of various drugs must be individually assessed with consideration given to the route of administration, the metabolic mechanism, and the presence of other competing drugs.

Changes in renal function

The most dramatic change with advancing age is a decrease in renal function. As a result, drugs that are excreted by glomerular filtration or active tubular secretion are removed more slowly and less completely. Glomerular filtration and renal tubular secretion decline with age by approximately 1% each year over the age of 40, so that the mean glomerular filtration rate of a normal adult aged 80 is approximately 60% of the rate at 40 years of age. In addition, reduction in renal blood flow and in glomerular filtration rate occurs as a result of various disease states such as congestive heart failure and dehydration.

Serum creatinine does not rise in proportion to the fall in renal function because reduced muscle mass produces less creatinine. Lowered creatinine clearance has been well documented in the older population even in the presence of normal serum creatinine. Therefore creatinine clearance is the critical variable in determining drug dosage in older adults with impaired renal function. Nomograms are published to estimate true creatinine clearance in relation to age. Decreased renal clearance may cause increased plasma drug concentrations and longer half-lives for drugs and active metabolites that are eliminated by the kidney. Special precautions are necessary when drugs of this type are administered to the elderly to monitor activity and decrease the risk of toxicity.

SUGGESTED READINGS

Bioavailability of drug products, Washington, D.C., 1975, American Pharmaceutical Association.

Evans, W., and others, editors: Applied principles of drug monitoring, San Francisco, 1980, Applied Therapeutics, Inc.

Ritschel, W.: Handbook of basic pharmacokinetics, ed. 2, Hamilton, Ill., 1980, Drug Intelligence Publications.

Winter, M.: Basic clinical pharmacokinetics, San Francisco, 1980, Applied Therapeutics, Inc.

GERIATRIC DRUG INTERACTIONS

4

Drug interaction is the phenomenon that occurs when the action of one drug is modified by the concurrent or subsequent administration of another drug. Drug interactions are frequently the causative factor of adverse drug reactions. Considerable attention has been given to the subject of drug interactions in recent years, and a number of comprehensive references deal exclusively with this subject. However, the clinical significance of many reported drug interactions is often obscure, and data about the magnitude of the problem in aging patients are frequently not available. As new, therapeutically effective drugs are introduced, more possibilities exist for the production of drug-related problems. It is important to understand how drugs interact to evaluate drug regimens and recognize the potential for interaction. It is also important that complete patient medication records be kept to prevent drug interaction problems from occurring or detect them early. The role of the pharmacist in monitoring drug therapy, suggesting modifications in drug regimens or elimination of unneeded drugs to other members of the health-care team or, when appropriate, to the patient, cannot be overemphasized.

FACTORS AFFECTING DRUG INTERACTIONS IN OLDER PERSONS

Two factors predispose the geriatric population to increased risk of complication from drug therapy: (1) physiological changes that produce alterations in the way drugs affect the body and (2) the need for multiple-drug therapy to treat a variety of disease states. It has been reported that the risk of drug reactions in adults 60 to 70 years of age is double that of those 30 to 40 years old. The aging process leads to an increase in disease states such as hypertension, diabetes, arthritis, heart failure, glaucoma, ulcers and other gastrointestinal problems, and urinary tract infections.

The treatment of these diseases leads to multiple-drug therapy or what is commonly known as polypharmacy, or polyprescribing by physicians. The more drugs a patient takes into the body, the greater the chances for adverse drug reactions. Physiological changes that occur in older adults affect the metabolism of drugs by the liver and the excretion of drugs by the kidney.

The major effect of these changes is to decrease the ability to compensate for interactions in which one drug affects the absorption, distribution, metabolism, or elimination of a second drug. Changes in tissue distribution and plasma protein binding of drugs make older adults more susceptible to displacement interactions and increase the difficulty of monitoring therapy effectively by using serum drug concentration measurements.

Age-related changes in receptor sensitivity have been suggested as the basis for both the increased and decreased response to some drugs in aging patients. Such changes in sensitivity could lead to a higher incidence of adverse drug reactions because of drug interaction.

Another factor influencing drug response is the inadequacy of homeostatic mechanisms to provide the control systems seen in younger patients. For example, the hypotension caused by combinations of antihypertensive drugs is much less effectively compensated for in older patients than in younger ones.

Other factors predisposing aging patients to drug interactions include the prescribing of usual doses of drugs without concern for altered physiology, the need for long-term administration of drugs that often have narrow therapeutic indexes, and the prescribing of drugs by multiple physicians. In addition, older patients are more assertive in exercising their right to treat themselves with nonprescription, over-the-counter drugs—preparations that may contribute to interactions between drugs. Self-administration of drugs by the elderly also increases the risks of interactions because of dose omissions, combining doses, and other errors of noncompliance.

The possibility of drug interaction developing should be considered in perspective. In many instances, two drugs known to interact can be administered concurrently as long as therapy is closely monitored and dosage adjustments are made to compensate for the altered response. Even if an altered response is predicted, it may not be of clinical significance in many patients, and, rather than omitting the therapeutic benefit of the offending drug, it can be administered with careful monitoring. In other situations, choice of another drug is possible, with similar therapeutic properties and less risk of interaction.

Since some drug interactions are beneficial, a second drug may be deliberately prescribed to modify the effects of another. A frequently cited example of a beneficial interaction is the use of probenecid to increase serum levels and lengthen the activity of penicillin derivatives in the body. Another example is the use of an antiparkinsonian drug with phenothiazine antipsychotic drugs to reduce the extrapyramidal side effects produced by the phenothiazines. The use of antidotes in the treatment of poisoning is based on useful antagonistic effects.

Numerous drug interactions have been reported in the literature, but not all are of clinical significance. The clinical significance of any interaction is based on the potential for harm to the patient and the extent of documentation. For example, an interaction of major clinical significance is one that can produce harm and is well documented. An interaction of minor clinical significance occurs with low incidence, demonstrates little potential for harm, and is poorly documented. Each patient brings a number of variables to each situation, and these variables influence the activity of the drug and its ability to interact with other drugs. It is difficult to predict the severity of even well-documented drug interactions because of individual variations in drug metabolism, disease states, diet, and genetic and environmental factors.

The mechanisms of drug interaction can be divided into two groups: (1) pharmacokinetic interactions in which the absorption, distribution, metabolism, or elimination of a drug is changed, and (2) pharmacodynamic interactions in which the pharmacological action of one drug is altered by the concurrent or subsequent administration of another drug. This group includes drugs having opposing or similar actions and drugs that alter receptor sensitivity.

We will discuss examples of each of these groups, using drugs frequently prescribed for geriatric patients. It must be recognized that more comprehensive reference sources, such as *Drug Interactions* by Hansten and *Evaluations of Drug Interactions*, published by the American Pharmaceutical Association, need to be used to provide additional information in the management of specific patient problems. Other sources of current drug information include the FDA-approved package insert and the professional service department of the pharmaceutical company that manufactures the drug.

PHARMACOKINETIC INTERACTIONS
Drug interactions altering absorption

The following are mechanisms of action that influence the absorption of a drug from the gastrointestinal tract.

Alteration of pH

Because many drugs are weak acids or weak bases and are present in solution both as nonionized and ionized forms, the pH of the gastrointestinal tract influences the site and extent of drug absorption and thus drug action. The nonionized, more lipid-soluble form is more readily absorbed than the ionized form. For example, weak acids such as barbiturates and aspirin are almost entirely nonionized in the stomach and well absorbed into the capillary blood. Weak bases such as morphine and quinine are highly ionized in gastric juice and poorly absorbed. Quinidine excretion is decreased as urinary pH increases. Because antacids can raise urinary pH, dangerous accumulation of quinidine is possible when the two drugs are concurrently administered. It can thus be predicted that antacid therapy will delay or partially prevent absorption of certain acidic drugs and enhance absorption of certain basic drugs. However, studies of the interactions of various drugs with antacids do not document significant clinical implication.

An interaction that should be noted here is that of bisacodyl and antacids. Bisacodyl is enteric coated because the drug is irritating. If it is administered within an hour of antacids or milk, an increase in the pH of the gastrointestinal contents may cause the enteric coating to disintegrate in the stomach, releasing the drug and causing irritation and vomiting.

Complexation

An example of complexation is the interaction between tetracycline and metal ions. The absorption of orally administered tetracyclines is decreased by antacids containing divalent or trivalent cations (e.g., calcium, magnesium, aluminum) because of the formation of poorly absorbed complexes. Iron salts cause the same type of interaction. Problems are avoided by separating administration of the two drugs by a minimum of 1 to 2 hours.

Cholestyramine and colestipol are used to complex with bile acids but also interfere with the absorption of other drugs because of the same binding mechanism. To minimize the possibility of this interaction, 4 to 5 hours should elapse between administration of these drugs and another drug having acidic properties.

Antidiarrheal mixtures (kaolin-pectin) and antacids can decrease absorption of other drugs such as phenothiazines and digoxin because of surface adsorptive properties. When reduced effects from drug therapy occur, attention should be given to the concurrent use of these mixtures causing altered absorption. Because digoxin is often poorly absorbed by older adults, any product that might further decrease its absorption could have significant adverse clinical effects. Taking the digoxin at least 1 hour apart from the other drugs will minimize the problem.

Change in rate of gastric emptying

By decreasing the rate of gastric emptying, anticholinergics such as propantheline, benztropine, and trihexyphenidyl influence drug absorption. Reduced peristalsis may slow dissolution, resulting in decreased absorption. However, the decrease in gastrointestinal motility also lengthens the time in which a drug can be absorbed, resulting in higher serum concentrations for many drugs, including digoxin. In addition to increasing gastric pH, antacids delay gastric emptying, producing varied effects in the absorption of drugs administered simultaneously.

The absorption of drugs is also influenced by food. Food reduces absorption of some drugs by slowing gastric emptying, decreasing the dissolution rate, and binding with drugs. Food may also increase absorption of selected drugs by delaying gastric emptying or by producing an increase in hepatic blood flow that reduces first-pass metabolism. To minimize variations in drug bioavailability caused by food, drug administration should be standardized in relationship to meals.

Drug interactions altering distribution

The distribution of drugs is achieved primarily by the blood plasma, which transports the drug to receptor sites and ultimately to excretion. Many drugs are not very soluble in plasma and are transported as complexes bound to plasma proteins such as albumin. This protein-bound fraction of a drug in the body is pharmacologically inert.

The drug action is due to the unbound or free drug at the receptor site, and therefore response to a drug is determined by the concentration of free drug in the plasma. As the unbound drug is metabolized and excreted, bound drug is released to maintain the pharmacological response. An interaction may occur when two drugs capable of binding to proteins are administered concurrently. If two drugs are given together or one after another, the drug more strongly bound remains tied to the protein-binding sites, and the less strongly bound drug is released into the plasma. The increase in plasma concentration causes an increase in the pharmacological activity, which may lead to undesirable effects. Drugs that are highly protein bound and subject to interactions include warfarin, phenylbutazone, barbiturates, phenytoin, salicylates, chloral hydrate, and sulfonamides. Because phenylbutazone displaces warfarin from plasma-binding sites, every effort should be made to avoid the use of phenylbutazone in patients receiving warfarin. Chloral hydrate may also potentiate the response to warfarin and is thus dangerous in combination with it. Disease states that influence drug-binding proteins, such as hypoalbuminemia or impaired renal function, may change the availability of drugs and increase the incidence of adverse effects.

Drug interactions altering metabolism

Biotransformation of drugs takes place mainly in the liver, where microsomal enzymes catalyze metabolic reactions, resulting in altered drug activity and more easily eliminated compounds. The microsomal enzymes involved in drug metabolism may be either stimulated or inhibited by the administration of drugs.

Enzyme stimulation

Enzyme stimulation, frequently referred to as enzyme induction, results in decreased drug activity because of an increased rate of metabolism and excretion. Most drugs are metabolized to less active metabolites. However, exceptions (such as the metabolizing of digitoxin to the active metabolite digoxin and meperidine to the toxic metabolite normeperidine) exist in which a drug may be converted to a more active metabolite, which may produce a greater clinical response than the parent compound. As a result of increased metabolism, increased doses are needed to maintain the desired activity.

When the drug that is producing the enzyme induction is withdrawn, a dangerous situation could arise unless the dose of the metabolized drug is also reduced. Phenobarbital is probably the best known example of the enzyme-stimulating drugs. The interaction that occurs when phenobarbital is administered to a patient receiving warfarin results in a decreased response to the anticoagulant because of the phenobarbital-induced enzyme activity producing more rapid metabolism and excretion of the warfarin. To compensate for the decrease in response, the dose of warfarin would have to be increased. If the phenobarbital were to be discontinued and the warfarin dose were not adjusted, there would be a risk of hemorrhage. Therefore barbiturate therapy should not be started or stopped without careful adjustment of the anticoagulant dose. When possible, a non-enzyme-inducing therapeutic alternative to the barbiturate should be used, such as flurazepam or diazepam. Other drugs that stimulate drug metabolism include hypnotics, anticonvulsants, antihistamines, sulfonylureas, and analgesics.

Stimulation of enzyme activity may also be responsible for the development of tolerance to certain drugs following chronic use. Larger doses are necessary to maintain the therapeutic effect because of the production of less active compounds resulting from enzymatic action.

Enzyme inhibition

Enzyme inhibition causes increased activity and prolonged action of some drugs. By inhibiting the enzyme xanthine oxidase, allopurinol produces a reduction in uric acid in the treatment of gout. Xanthine oxidase is the enzyme involved in the metabolism of mercaptopurine and azathioprine. When allopurinol is given in combination with either mercaptopurine or azathioprine, a reduction in dose of about one third to one fourth is required for these antineoplastic drugs. This example illustrates the possibility of an increased response to the drug whose metabolism has been inhibited unless the combination is avoided or recognized in advance and necessary precautions taken. Cimetidine affects microsomal enzyme systems, which reduces hepatic metabolism. This mechanism delays elimination and elevates blood levels of many drugs, including propranolol, diazepam, theophylline, phenytoin, and coumarin.

Drug interactions altering renal excretion

Influencing the excretion of one drug by another through the kidney can increase or decrease drug action. Interactions altering renal excretion can occur through change in the urine pH or by interference with transport systems in the kidney cells. Renal function is one of the most important factors determining drug activity.

Reduced renal function in the older adult leads to adverse drug reactions because of slower rates of excretion, producing increased drug plasma levels. Significant drug interactions could result when a patient is taking a combination of drugs excreted by the kidney. Doses of drugs such as the digitalis glycosides and aminoglycoside antibiotics need to be adjusted downward in patients with reduced renal function to avoid toxic reactions.

The renal clearance of acidic drugs is increased in alkaline urine and decreased in acid urine. The opposite is true for basic drugs, which are excreted more quickly from acidic urine and more slowly from alkaline urine. Changes in urinary pH can occur because of chronic administration of antacids, acidifying agents such as methenamine and ascorbic acid, alkalinizing agents such as sodium bicarbonate, and various foods. Large doses, in the range of 12 g/day, of ascorbic acid or vitamin C are needed to acidify the urine sufficiently to be effective. Unless the dose is adequate, the use of this drug for this purpose should be questioned. Salicylate plasma levels are influenced by changes in urinary pH, especially in patients using large doses for arthritic conditions. As urinary pH decreases, salicylate plasma levels increase, and this increase could produce toxic symptoms.

The excretion of drugs that are actively secreted or reabsorbed by tubular cells can be blocked by other drugs competing for the same transport mechanism. By inhibiting the penicillin transport mechanism in the kidney, probenecid increases serum levels and prolongs the activity of penicillin derivatives.

In the same way, salicylates can inhibit the activity of probenecid and other uricosuric agents. A reduction in the renal clearance of digoxin is induced by the concurrent administration of quinidine. To reduce the possibility of toxic effects occurring from the increased serum concentrations of digoxin, a reduction of half the maintenance dose is recommended in patients with normal renal function when quinidine is administered concurrently. Routine monitoring of serum digoxin levels will help the physician assess therapy when both drugs are employed.

PHARMACODYNAMIC INTERACTIONS

The concurrent or sequential administration of two or more drugs having similar pharmacological effects or side effects may cause drug interactions because of the additive effect of these properties. The most obvious examples of this type of interaction involve the administration of CNS depressants such as sedatives, hypnotics, tranquilizers, analgesics, anticonvulsants, and antipsychotic drugs. Often this depressant effect is potentiated by the consumption of alcoholic beverages. It is extremely important that the patient be cautioned about the use of alcohol while taking CNS depressant drugs. In addition, the patient needs to be warned about the effects of these drugs and alcohol on various motor skills such as driving and advised to exercise caution while using household or job-related equipment.

Many drugs commonly used in the care of geriatric patients possess anticholinergic activity, which causes side effects such as dryness of the mouth, blurred vision, urinary retention, constipation, and increased intraocular pressure. Antiparkinsonian drugs, antidepressants, antipsychotic drugs, and antihistamines all contribute to this type of complication. Excessive anticholinergic activity can cause an atropine-like delirium often mistaken for an increase in psychiatric symptoms in the elderly patient. This condition may be erroneously treated by increasing the dose of an antipsychotic drug, which would only add to the problem.

Drugs having opposing pharmacological effects also cause interactions by reducing the clinical effects of other concurrently administered drugs. Overly sedating drugs may be given with stimulants, and small doses of sedatives may be given with stimulating drugs to reduce the unwanted effect. Timolol, a β-adrenergic blocking agent used topically to treat glaucoma, can cause the loss of control of previously stabilized asthmatic patients on β-adrenergic drugs such as terbutaline. Orally administered drugs with anticholinergic activity may interfere with the action of a topically administered cholinergic drug such as pilocarpine.

Alterations in electrolyte levels of ions such as potassium, sodium, calcium, and magnesium can also result in a drug interaction. The excessive loss of potassium produced by most diuretics causes a predisposition to digitalis toxicity. The potassium deficiency may be corrected by supplementing the diet with foods rich in potassium, taking a pharmaceutical potassium supplement, or using a potassium-sparing diuretic in combination with the potassium-depleting agent. Diuretics also cause magnesium deficiencies, which contribute to the problem with digitalis drugs. Potassium depletion can also be caused by long-term use of laxatives and corticosteroids. Overuse of laxative products is common in our older population, since good health is equated with regular bowel movements. Elderly patients frequently have inadequate diets, which further complicate diagnosis and therapy. Sodium loss increases the activity of lithium and may lead to toxicity unless dosage adjustments are made. Patients receiving diuretic therapy or on sodium-restricted diets should not receive lithium unless therapeutic alternatives are not available.

Further possibilities for drug interactions occur with guanethidine and monoamine oxidase (MAO) inhibitors. Both tricyclic antidepressants and antipsychotic drugs inhibit the uptake of guanethidine into the adrenergic neuron, and this inhibition results in the reversal of guanethidine's antihypertensive effects. Sympathomimetic drugs such as ephedrine, phenylephrine, and phenylpropanolamine are metabolized by monoamine oxidase. When this enzyme is inhibited, norepinephrine levels increase in the adrenergic neuron. The concurrent administration of sympathomimetic drugs results in the release of a large amount of norepinephrine. Severe reactions occur, including hypertensive crisis and cardiac arrhythmias.

Another frequently overlooked area that contributes to the possibilities for drug interaction is self-medication for self-limited symptoms not requiring medical supervision. The use of nonprescription medication, referred to as over-the-counter medication, is common in today's society and is recognized as an essential part of health care. Effective self-care by the patient reduces the load on the health-care system and contributes to the individual's assessment and management of common health problems.

Important components of self-medication include recognition of the symptoms for which self-medication is appropriate, selection of the proper over-the-counter product, and administration of the selected product according to labeled directions. Equally important is the person's ability to recognize the need to seek medical advice if symptoms are not alleviated within an adequate time. Over-the-counter drugs are considered relatively safe if used according to labeled directions, but the use of these drugs is not without potential risk, especially in the older population. Small print on the bottle may lead to difficulty in understanding labeled directions. Excessive use may lead to overdose and toxicity. Even if the drug is used according to labeled directions, adverse drug reactions may occur because of alterations in physiology or hypersensitivity. Drug interactions can occur between two or more over-the-counter products used concurrently as well as the multiple prescription medications used in the medical management of the geriatric patient.

Of the multitude of over-the-counter products available for selection and self-administration, the most commonly used preparations are the following: (1) aspirin and aspirin-containing preparations used for acute or chronic pain, (2) sympathomimetic amines and antihistamines used to provide relief from nasal stuffiness that is due to colds and allergic rhinitis, (3) antacids used to treat acid indigestion, sour stomach, and heartburn, (4) laxatives to maintain expected patterns of regular bowel movements, and (5) antidiarrheal preparations to treat diarrhea and associated symptoms of gastrointestinal upset.

GUIDELINES TO DECREASE DRUG INTERACTIONS

An awareness of the more important drug interactions and knowledge of the mechanisms of drug interactions can help avoid or minimize adverse drug reactions or ineffective treatment from multiple drug therapy. Guidelines to assist the professional in this area of responsibility include the following:

1. Take a careful drug history from the patient of both prescribed and self-administered drugs.
2. Avoid multiple-drug therapy when possible.
3. When multiple-drug therapy is indicated, minimize interactions by taking advantage of pharmacokinetic and pharmacological factors such as sequence of administration, route and time of administration, duration of therapy, dose adjustments, substitution of safer drugs with similar action, and use of a different dosage form.
4. Avoid unnecessary changes in drug therapy.
5. Observe therapy carefully when using drugs known to cause significant clinical interactions.
6. Instruct the patient in the possible risks and action to follow when using drug combinations with interaction potential.

In summary, the key to preventing drug interactions is to be aware of such possibilities whenever more than one drug is being administered, when switching from one drug to another, when discontinuing one or more drugs, and when carefully assessing the patient's physiological state before prescribing.

The following boxed material provides a summary of interaction information involving therapeutic agents most frequently prescribed for geriatric patients. More comprehensive information may be obtained from previously listed resources.

GERIATRIC DRUG INTERACTIONS*

ANALGESICS

Salicylates with

Alcohol	Occult blood loss from salicylates may be increased. Risk of gastrointestinal hemorrhage is increased.
Antacids	Serum salicylate levels in patients taking large doses of aspirin are decreased.
Anticoagulants (oral)	Anticoagulant effects may increase, especially with large doses of aspirin. There is also a possibility of gastrointestinal ulceration, impaired primary hemostasis, and hemorrhage.
Antidiabetics	Hypoglycemic response may increase, especially in patients taking sulfonylureas and moderate to large doses of aspirin.
Corticosteroids	Blood salicylate levels are decreased; when both drugs are taken together, salicylism may result if the corticosteroid dose is reduced. There is also additive ulcerogenic potential.
Fenoprofen	Fenoprofen activity may be reduced.
Indomethacin	Indomethacin blood levels may be reduced. There is also additive ulcerogenic potential.
Methotrexate	Methotrexate toxicity may be increased.
Naproxen	Naproxen activity may be reduced.
Phenytoin	Large doses of salicylates potentiate the activity of phenytoin by displacing it from plasma protein-binding sites.
Probenecid	Aspirin in low doses inhibits uricosuric activity of probenecid.
Sulfinpyrazone	Aspirin inhibits uricosuric activity of sulfinpyrazone.

---

*Interactions designated in italics are relatively well documented and have harmful potential to the patient.

Continued.

GERIATRIC DRUG INTERACTIONS—cont'd

ANTICOAGULANTS

Coumarin anticoagulants (warfarin) with

Aspirin and other salicylates	Anticoagulant effect is increased. Substitute acetaminophen unless antiinflammatory action is needed.
Antacids	Anticoagulant effect may be decreased. Separate administration times by 1-2 hr.
Antidepressants	Anticoagulant effect may be increased. It may be necessary to decrease warfarin dose.
Barbiturates	Anticoagulant effect is decreased. In a patient taking both drugs, hemorrhage may occur if the barbiturate is discontinued without warfarin dose reduction. Substitute benzodiazepine for barbiturate if possible.
Chloral hydrate	Anticoagulant effect may be increased.
Cholestyramine Colestipol	Absorption may be decreased. Give warfarin 1 hr before or 4-6 hr after cholestyramine/colestipol administration.
Phenylbutazone Oxyphenbutazone	Anticoagulant effect and risk of gastrointestinal bleeding are increased. Avoid concurrent use. Substitute tolmetin.
Phenytoin	Anticoagulant effect is decreased, and phenytoin effect is increased.
Quinidine	Anticoagulant effect is increased. It may be necessary to decrease quinidine dose or substitute procainamide.
Rifampin	Anticoagulant effect is decreased.
Sulfonylurea hypoglycemic agents	Hypoglycemic effect is increased.
Vitamin K	Use as antidote for warfarin overdose. Avoid excessive use of vitamin K–containing drugs or foods (e.g., green leafy vegetables) and liquid nutritional products containing vitamin K, such as Ensure.

GERIATRIC DRUG INTERACTIONS—cont'd

ANTIHISTAMINES

Antihistamines with

Alcohol	Combined use results in additive CNS depression.
Anticholinergics Atropine Dicyclomine Glycopyrrolate Isopropamide Propantheline Trihexyphenidyl	Combined use results in additive sedation and enhanced atropine-like effects.
Antidepressants Amitriptyline Amoxapine Desipramine Doxepin Imipramine Maprotiline Nortriptyline Protriptyline Trazodone	Combined use results in enhanced atropine-like effect.
CNS Depressants Sedatives Narcotics	Combined use results in additive CNS depression.
Hormones Estradiol Prednisone Testosterone	Effectiveness of the hormone may be reduced because of the antihistamine's ability to induce hepatic microsomal enzymes.

ANTIPSYCHOTIC AGENTS

Phenothiazines and haloperidol with

Antacids	Antipsychotic response is decreased.
Anticholinergics	Extrapyramidal effects are decreased.
Antihypertensives	Hypotensive effect is increased.
Guanethidine	Hypotensive effect is decreased.
Levodopa	Control of parkinsonism is decreased. Avoid concurrent use if possible.
MAO inhibitors	Extrapyramidal effects are increased.

Continued.

GERIATRIC DRUG INTERACTIONS—cont'd

ANTIPSYCHOTIC AGENTS—cont'd

Lithium with

NOTE: Lithium is contraindicated for patients on salt-restricted diets because of possible toxicity.

Diuretics	Increased excretion of sodium may result in increased retention of lithium and possible toxicity.
Potassium iodide	Hypothyroid activity is increased.
Sodium chloride	Lithium response is decreased.

CARDIOVASCULAR AGENTS

Cardiac glycosides (e.g., digoxin) with

Antacids	Digoxin effect is decreased.
Anticholinergic agents	Digoxin effect is increased.
Antidiarrheal adsorbents	Digoxin effect is decreased.
Cholestyramine Colestipol	Absorption of digoxin is decreased. Give digoxin 1 hr before or 4-6 hr after cholestyramine/colestipol administration.
Diuretics, potassium-depleting	Absorption of digoxin is decreased. Give digoxin 1 hr before or 4-6 hr after diuretic administration.
Quinidine	Serum digoxin levels increase and may produce toxicity. Decrease digoxin dose by 50% at the start of quinidine therapy and monitor serum digoxin concentrations to adjust dose.

Propranolol with

Aminophylline and theophylline derivatives	Effects of both drugs are inhibited. If aminophylline is being used to treat asthma, propranolol should be avoided.
Furosemide Hydralazine Chlorpromazine Cimetidine	Antihypertensive effect is increased. Dosage adjustment may be required.
Hypoglycemic agents	Hypoglycemic effect may be increased.
Indomethacin	Antihypertensive effect is reduced.

GERIATRIC DRUG INTERACTIONS—cont'd

Reserpine with

Digoxin	Risk of cardiac arrhythmias is increased.
Levodopa	Levodopa effect is reduced. Avoid combination.
Tricyclic antidepressants	Reserpine should be withdrawn if causing depression.

Antihypertensive drugs with

Diuretics Other antihypertensive drugs Phenothiazines Tricyclic antidepressants Vasodilators	Hypotensive effect is increased. Adequate control may be achieved with lower doses.

Guanethidine with

Alcohol	Hypotensive effect is increased. Avoid or limit alcohol intake.
Phenothiazines	Hypotensive effect is reduced.
Reserpine	Combination may produce excessive orthostatic hypotension, bradycardia, and depression.
Tricyclic antidepressants	Antihypertensive effect is inhibited. Drug substitution is required.

Methyldopa with

Levodopa	Effects of both agents are increased. Dose adjustments may be required.

DIURETICS

Potassium-depleting diuretics with

Digoxin	Risk of digitalis toxicity is increased. Potassium replacement may be required.
Lithium	Combination increases lithium effects and toxicity. If possible, avoid drug combination.
Hypoglycemic agents	Blood glucose is increased. Dose adjustment may be required.

Continued.

GERIATRIC DRUG INTERACTIONS—cont'd

DIURETICS—cont'd

Spironolactone and triamterene with

Potassium chloride	Combining drugs may cause hyperkalemia. Avoid drug combination.

GASTROINTESTINAL AGENTS

Antacids with

Bisacodyl	Combination may cause gastrointestinal irritation because of disintegration of the enteric coating and release of the bisacodyl in the stomach. Separate administration times by 1 hr.
Digoxin	Absorption of digoxin is decreased.
Iron preparations	Magnesium trisilicate decreases absorption of iron.
Isoniazid	Absorption of isoniazid is decreased. Separate administration times by 1 hr.
Phenothiazines	Plasma levels of the phenothiazine are decreased. Separate administration times by 1 hr.
Quinidine	Antacids increase renal tubular reabsorption of quinidine, which increases urinary pH.
Salicylates	Antacids may decrease serum salicylate levels in patients taking large doses of aspirin by reducing renal tubular reabsorption.
Tetracyclines	Tetracycline activity is decreased because of chelation with divalent or trivalent cations. Separate administration times by 1-2 hr.

Cimetidine with

Anticoagulants	Anticoagulant effect is increased. Monitor response to oral anticoagulants when cimetidine is started or stopped or dose is changed.
Benzodiazepines	Response to many benzodiazepines is increased (exceptions are lorazepam and oxazepam).
Phenytoin	Serum phenytoin levels are increased. Bone marrow suppression is possible.
Propranolol	Propranolol-induced bradycardia is increased.

GERIATRIC DRUG INTERACTIONS—cont'd

Theophylline	Serum theophylline levels are increased. Combination may produce toxicity. Monitor theophylline serum levels.

HYPOGLYCEMICS

Sulfonylureas with

Corticosteroids	Blood glucose levels are increased. Dose of hypoglycemic agent may need to be increased.
Dextrothyroxine	Blood glucose levels are increased. Increase in dose of hypoglycemic agent may be needed.
Diuretics	Blood glucose levels are increased. Increase in dose of hypoglycemic agent may be needed.
Coumarin anticoagulants	Hypoglycemic effect is increased.
Phenylbutazone	Hypoglycemic effect is increased.
Propranolol	Combination may mask early signs and symptoms characteristic of acute hypoglycemia.

LAXATIVES

Bisacodyl with

Antacids	Combination may cause gastrointestinal irritation because of disintegration of the enteric coating and release of the bisacodyl in the stomach. Separate administration times by 1 hr.

Docusate with

Mineral oil	Absorption of mineral oil may be increased.

Mineral oil with

Anticoagulants Estrogens Sulfonamides Vitamin A	Absorption may be impaired.

Phospho-soda with

Isoniazid	Absorption may be impaired.

Continued.

GERIATRIC DRUG INTERACTIONS—cont'd

OVER-THE-COUNTER ORAL DECONGESTANTS

Phenylephrine with

Guanethidine	Antihypertensive effect of guanethidine is antagonized, and control of blood pressure may be lost.
Methyldopa	Antihypertensive effect of methyldopa is antagonized, and control of blood pressure may be lost.
MAO inhibitors	Combined use may produce increased hypertensive response, tachycardia, and arrhythmias.
Reserpine	Antihypertensive effect of reserpine is antagonized, and control of blood pressure may be lost.
Tricyclic antidepressants	Hypertensive response to phenylephrine is increased.

Phenylpropanolamine with

β-adrenergic blockers	Combined use may produce a severe hypertensive reaction.
MAO inhibitors	Combined use may produce increased hypertensive response, tachycardia, and arrhythmias.

Pseudoephedrine with

Kaolin	Pseudoephedrine absorption is reduced.
MAO inhibitors	Combined use may produce a severe hypertensive reaction. Avoid combination.

PSYCHOPHARMACOLOGICAL AGENTS

Psychopharmacological agents with

Alcohol	Depressant effect is increased. Avoid consumption of alcoholic beverages if possible.

Tricyclic antidepressants with

Antihypertensive agents	Antihypertensive effect is increased. Decrease in dose of antihypertensive agent may be needed.
Coumarin anticoagulants	Anticoagulant effect is increased. Decrease in dose of anticoagulant may be needed.
Guanethidine	Antihypertensive effect is decreased.

GERIATRIC DRUG INTERACTIONS—cont'd

MAO inhibitors	Concurrent use is contraindicated. Severe atropine-like reactions, convulsions, hyperpyrexia, and delirium have been reported.
Reserpine	Combination may cause depression. Concurrent use is contraindicated.

MAO inhibitors with

Alcohol	Hypertensive crisis may result if the alcoholic beverage contains tyramine.
Tricyclic antidepressants	Convulsions, hyperpyrexia, and other severe adverse effects are possible with concurrent use.
Barbiturates	Combination may enhance and prolong effects of barbiturates.
Ephedrine	Hypertension is possible with concurrent use.
Epinephrine	Combination may enhance epinephrine's effect.
Hypoglycemics	Combination may increase or prolong hypoglycemic response to insulin and oral agents.
Levodopa	Hypertension, flushing, palpitations, lightheadedness, worsening of akinesia, and tremor are possible with concurrent use. Carbidopa given with levodopa seems to prevent the interaction.
Meperidine	Excitation, sweating, rigidity, hypertension or hypotension, and coma are possible with concurrent use.
Phenylephrine	Hypertension is possible with concurrent use.
Phenylpropanolamine	Hypertension is possible with concurrent use.
Pseudoephedrine	Concurrent use may cause acute hypertensive effects in patients chronically receiving MAO inhibitors. Combination should be avoided.
Reserpine	Excitation and hypertension are possible with concurrent use.
Tyramine	Combination may cause severe hypertension. Substances containing tyramine include certain cheeses, alcoholic beverages, nuts, sour cream, pickled herring, chicken liver, broad beans, chocolate, and yeast extract. Tyramine is not available as such for any clinical purpose.

Continued.

GERIATRIC DRUG INTERACTIONS—cont'd

SEDATIVE-HYPNOTICS

Barbiturates with

Alcohol	Additive CNS depression is possible with concurrent use.
Anticoagulants	Response to anticoagulants is decreased. In a patient taking both drugs, hemorrhage may occur if the barbiturate is discontinued.
Tricyclic antidepressants	Antidepressant effect is reduced.
β-adrenergic blockers	β-adrenergic blocker effectiveness is reduced.
Corticosteroids	Effects of corticosteroid therapy (especially in steroid-dependent asthmatic patients) are reduced.
Griseofulvin	Therapeutic response to griseofulvin is impaired.
MAO inhibitors	Effects of barbiturates are enhanced.
Oral hypoglycemics	Hypoglycemic effect is reduced.
Phenytoin	Phenytoin intoxication may result when barbiturates are withdrawn from patients being maintained on both drugs.
Quinidine	Effectiveness of quinidine is reduced.

Chloral hydrate with

Alcohol	Concurrent use increases CNS depression, including impairment of motor function, flushing, tachycardia, and headache.
Anticoagulants	Hypoprothrombinemia is increased.

Benzodiazepines with

Alcohol	Concurrent use increases CNS depression.
Tricyclic antidepressants	Concurrent use enhances atropine-like effects.
Levodopa	Concurrent use of benzodiazepine may decrease control of parkinsonism by levodopa.
Phenytoin	Phenytoin toxicity is increased.

URICOSURICS

Allopurinol with

Anticoagulants	Anticoagulant effect is enhanced.
Antidiabetics	Hypoglycemic activity is enhanced.

GERIATRIC DRUG INTERACTIONS—cont'd

Azathioprine	Combined use may cause bone marrow depression.
Cyclophosphamide	Combination increases risk of bone marrow depression.
Mercaptopurine	Combined use increases both antineoplastic activity and toxic effects of mercaptopurine. Possible severe toxicity could result.
Probenecid	Combination inhibits metabolism of probenecid, causing possible toxicity from probenecid. Concurrent use also increases renal elimination of the active metabolite of allopurinol, creating possibility of reduced response to allopurinol.

Probenecid with

Allopurinol	Allopurinol appears to inhibit the metabolism of probenecid, causing possible toxicity from probenecid. Probenecid increases renal elimination of the active metabolite of allopurinol, creating the possibility of reduced response to allopurinol.
Cephalosporins	Combination increases the risk of nephrotoxicity from cephalosporins.
Indomethacin	Concurrent use enhances indomethacin activity.
Methotrexate	Combination may lead to elevated serum levels of methotrexate and increased risk of methotrexate toxicity.
Salicylates	Combined use may inhibit uricosuric activity of probenecid.
Sulfinpyrazone	Concurrent use may increase risk of toxicity with sulfinpyrazone.

Sulfinpyrazone with

Antidiabetics	Combination enhances hypoglycemic activity of oral hypoglycemic agents and insulin.
Probenecid	Concurrent use increases risk of toxicity with probenecid.
Salicylates	Each drug inhibits the uricosuric activity of the other.

REFERENCES

Evaluations of drug interactions, ed. 2, Washington, D.C., 1976, American Pharmaceutical Association.

Evaluations of drug interactions, supplement, Washington, D.C., 1978, American Pharmaceutical Association.

Hansten, P., editor: Drug interactions, ed. 4, Philadelphia, 1979, Lea & Febiger.

SUGGESTED READINGS

Bressler, R.: Understanding adverse drug reactions in the elderly, Drug Therapy **10:**73, 1981.

Lamy, P.: Drug interactions and the elderly: a new perspective, Drug Intell. Clin. Pharm. **14:**514, 1980.

Simonson, W.: Geriatric considerations for drug interactions, Pharmacy Times **47:**60, 1981.

5

MISUSE AND ABUSE OF MEDICATION

With increased public awareness of aging and associated problems, general interest in the drug habits of older adults has developed. The literature indicates that misuse of drugs by older adults is a serious problem demanding attention. Twenty-five percent of all prescription drugs are purchased by the older population group. Because of this large volume, possibility for misuse will be more common. Accurate statistics for over-the-counter drugs purchased by this population are unavailable, but because of the high incidence of chronic illness, an assumption can be made that they purchase a similar percentage of these products. Frequent usage of both prescribed and self-selected drugs increases the risk for drug misuse in the elderly population. This chapter will explore medication misuse and abuse, including the use of alcohol.

SELF-MEDICATION

Self-medication comprises two separate problems, self-treatment and self-administration, which will be discussed separately. Self-treatment is diagnosing a health problem, selecting a specific treatment, purchasing an over-the-counter medication, and taking this treatment without supervision. Self-administration is the administration of a medication that has been prescribed by a physician.

Self-diagnosis and treatment

There are numerous reasons why older adults diagnose their illnesses and prescribe their own treatment. Foremost among the reasons is the charge for a physician visit combined with the cost of the prescribed drug. The fee for an office visit may or may not be paid by a third party. Unfortunately, older persons on fixed incomes may not be aware of, or be too proud to go to, a health center or clinic where they can receive the type of care they need for a lower cost. Delay in getting an appointment can be frustrating. The health problem is perceived as one of urgency, and then it is learned that it will be necessary to wait several weeks, or possibly an appointment is refused because requirements are not met. If an appointment is made, the person may have a problem reaching the practitioner's office because of restricted activity or lack of transportation. A frequent situation encountered by older persons is the lack of a personal physician; the prior physician has retired, moved away, or died; or perhaps the person has never had a personal physician. Regardless, there is no practitioner available to the person for diagnosis and treatment.

Fear is another reason why people do not seek appropriate treatment from qualified practitioners. The concern is for the possible diagnosis—cancer, high blood pressure, diabetes? A symptom that may have been minimized previously now becomes more apparent, but persons are afraid to seek help because of the possible diagnosis or the preconceived constraints that prescribed treatment may have on their life-style.

The influence of family and friends may also be a reason the older persons do not seek appropriate care. They learn from this group the possible cause of the problem and remedies that they have found effective. Advertising also makes them aware of possible causes and treatments that are available without prescription. A proliferation of available literature may clarify or cloud the person's perception of the problem or treatment.

Making the diagnosis

What kinds of problems may the person be diagnosing? The National Council on Aging (1978) reported that the five most prevalent chronic conditions affecting the aged are arthritis, hearing impairment, vision impairment, hypertension, and heart disease. Additional problems reported by Lofholm (1978) were digestive diseases, chronic sinusitis, mental and nervous disorders, genitourinary problems, and circulatory problems. The consumer lacks the factual knowledge to recognize the real problem while symptoms are treated, and the original problem may become more serious.

Selecting the treatment

How does a person make a choice regarding self-prescribed treatment? The media, including radio, television, newspapers, and magazines, are very influential, especially when special offers are made for drugs commonly used by older people. The presence of an older person in the advertisement also influences the choice of treatment. The availability of over-the-counter, or nonprescription, drugs in pharmacies, discount houses, supermarkets, and mail-order houses makes purchase relatively easy.

Over-the-counter medications commonly purchased by older adults include antacids, analgesics, laxatives, antiinflammatory agents, cough medicines, nasal decongestants, and topical skin preparations. Older friends with similar conditions may advise treatment or share their medicine for a trial. The placement of the product with other desirable products commonly used by older adults within the pharmacy is a factor in making the choice. The packaging may proclaim success in treating the present symptoms.

Another factor influencing choice of treatment is success with previous treatment. The person may have had a seemingly similar problem and decides to use the medication that had been previously prescribed or that had been purchased without a prescription.

On a more positive side, older adults may seek help from a health-care provider, either a nurse or pharmacist. Current preparation of these practitioners includes skills in health assessment, broad-based clinical knowledge, and also an awareness of changes that occur with aging. Practitioners should proceed with caution in advising treatment because of the complexity of multiple illnesses, potential drug interactions and side effects when a variety of medications are taken, and the general vulnerability of the older population. The legality of such advice should be investigated through appropriate professional literature and organizations.

Potential problems with self-treatment

The most obvious problem related to self-treatment is an incorrect diagnosis. The fatigue that a person has been treating with large doses of vitamins was caused by hypoxia. The ankle edema that the person was treating with herbal tea or magnesium sulfate soaks was caused by congestive heart failure. These examples emphasize the fact that correct diagnosis requires a high level of skill that the consumer does not possess. In both these situations proper treatment was delayed as the condition worsened.

Another problem concerns the interaction of the self-prescribed drug with other drugs the person is taking. Most persons perceive over-the-counter drugs as safe and effective, but in actuality they can be dangerous. Antacids can affect the use of multiple drugs such as digitalis, tetracyclines, phenothiazines, quinidine, and iron. Consuming alcohol with sedatives, antidepressants, antipsychotics, and antihistamines can have deleterious effects.

Because several illnesses may occur simultaneously in one person, self-prescribed treatment for one condition may be harmful to another. The laxative may have a high sodium content, which can further complicate existing circulatory problems. The cough medicine may be high in sugar content, further complicating proper control of diabetes. When self-diagnosing and prescribing, persons may not be aware of conditions that may exist in their own bodies for which the self-prescribed medications are used with caution. For example, they may not be aware of hypertension that is becoming more critical with the use of nasal decongestants and antihistamines.

Drugs used for the previous treatment of a similar condition may be hazardous because the condition may not actually be the same or the medication may have deteriorated. Certain drugs, such as nitroglycerin, eye drops, and antibiotic suspensions, deteriorate and become less effective when improperly stored, or decomposition may cause unexpected side effects.

In addition to the preceding problems associated with self-treatment, the patient does not readily report self-treatment to the physician. This lack of reporting may be innocent, because an over-the-counter drug may not be viewed by the patient as a form of treatment. When taking a history, the examiner must ask the patient about previous symptoms and any kind of treatment that might have been used. Examples of treatment may be necessary to obtain a full history.

In summary, people are more knowledgeable regarding illness and more resources are available, but older persons must be cautioned against self-diagnosis and treatment without adequate knowledge and supervision. Pharmacists, nurses, and other health professionals, who have an understanding of the effects of the aging process and who thoroughly assess the patient's situation, can help the person determine possible therapy and referral to a physician as necessary. Management of minor aches and pains with over-the-counter medication can prove successful, providing that the patient has access to reliable information.

Self-administration

The earlier portion of this chapter dealt with self-treatment, or the self-diagnosing and self-prescribing of medications. This section will deal with self-administration, which is defined as the administration of a prescription drug that has been prescribed by a physician or licensed health professional who has been approved for this function. Self-administration is usually carried out independently but may be supervised by a practitioner such as a public health nurse.

Because 95% of older adults live in the community, they presumably manage their own medication. It is projected that by the year 2000, 33 million older adults will be managing their own medication regimen, creating the potential for significant misuse.

The literature regarding self-administration among the elderly places major focus on compliance, or the ability to adhere to the therapeutic regimen. In a classic study of elderly, chronically ill ambulatory patients, Schwartz (1975) found that approximately half the group of patients had made medication errors. Medication errors followed a similar pattern. Most frequent were errors of omission, followed by inappropriate self-medication. Incorrect dose, improper timing, and inaccurate knowledge of the drug were three additional, frequently appearing errors. Lundin (1978), in a study of older persons living in the community, found that frequent causes of errors were inadequate knowledge of medications and insufficient direction in taking medication. Others have written about the necessity of developing concern for medication use among the independent elderly who are responsible for their own medication decisions, since many adverse medication reactions and interactions can be prevented. Lofholm (1978) points out that with sufficient knowledge, medications can control chronic illness, permitting an independent life-style for many older adults.

Factors affecting compliance

A variety of factors can affect the patient's ability to comply with the prescribed regimen. When a patient leaves the physician's office with a prescription, it is assumed that the prescription will be filled and the medication taken. However, this does not always occur. The practitioner may have failed to emphasize the importance of the therapy, and as a result, the prescription may not have been filled. Patients may not have understood the diagnosis or may not wish to improve their condition. In some circumstances, the therapy is affected by their general health beliefs, or they may not wish to relinquish the sick role if it has previously produced worthwhile gains.

Inability to understand specific instructions. The practitioner may fail to give instructions in a clear, specific manner. Because patient education may not be a priority in professional practice, or perhaps because of other pressures, instructions are not slowly and clearly articulated. The labeling on the container may be in small print with some instructions vague, especially the time for administration, which is often unclear on the label. A case in point is the container labeled "take one or two tablets p.r.n. for pain." A prescription of this type requires a high degree of judgment from the patient. When should one tablet or two tablets be taken, and how frequently can they be taken?

Complexity of regimen. Because of the multiple health problems encountered by older adults, therapeutic regimens may become very complex, with three to twelve medications prescribed simultaneously (Lamy, 1980). The variety and number of medications, doses, and times of administration greatly affect compliance. At a time in life when problem-solving skills begin to falter, the older person is expected to make decisions about a complex plan.

A common concern is how the medication should be taken—with food, without food, with milk, with certain kinds of juices, or with a full glass of water. If the patient is unable to swallow the medication, can it be divided, crushed, or dissolved, or is it available in liquid form? Confusion also may occur about whether a medication should be chewed, swallowed whole, or dissolved in the mouth. Explicit instructions are necessary.

Anyone can become confused about the time to take medications with a complicated regimen. Common concerns are: Is it best to take the medication before, with, or after meals? Is it best to take daily medications in the morning or evening? Is it safe to change the time of taking a diuretic to make a social engagement more enjoyable? These are questions commonly asked. It has been demonstrated that compliance increases if the frequency of taking the medications decreases. When consulting with patients regarding their total medication schedules, the nurse should discuss alterations to simplify the regimen.

Lack of knowledge about medications. Patients have a right to know what they can expect from a drug, including the expected action, the side effects that can occur, the precautions and hazards associated with taking the drug, other drugs that are to be avoided because of interactions that may occur, and the dangers of noncompliance. The appearance of side effects when there has been no previous warning can be very disturbing to older adults and is often a reason for discontinuing the medication. Practitioners do not agree about what patients should be told about side effects, but this lack of knowledge can also be responsible for developing mistrust in the patient-practitioner relationship. Patients may feel that the side effects are worse than the original problem. Would they prefer to have the discomforts of arthritis rather than the gastric distress of aspirin, or the restlessness of anxiety rather than the drowsiness caused by diazepam? These are decisions patients make when not given information about side effects. Informing patients about common side effects and indicating what action to take if they occur can promote compliance.

Nature of the disease. The nature of the disease is also a factor. Noncompliance is most likely with mild and chronic disorders that require prophylactic or suppressive therapy and diseases in which the consequences of stopping therapy may be delayed. Hypertension is a classic example. When the person is asymptomatic, does not understand the need for continued treatment, and discontinues therapy or decreases the dose, the consequences may not be manifest until later.

Fear of drug dependency. The emphasis in the media on the causes and hazards of drug dependency are concerns of older adults and a cause of noncompliance. Peers may depend on psychoactive drugs that are affecting their behavior, and this effect can be frightening. To diminish the possibility of dependency, they may omit or substitute over-the-counter drugs that are less effective.

Medication dose forms. Medications that are difficult to prepare or measure or have an unpleasant taste, odor, or appearance may also be disregarded by the older adult. Offering suggestions about how to camouflage the taste or discussing with the physician an alternative form of medication that is more palatable can promote compliance. For measurement problems, perhaps unit dose–packaged drugs may be the answer.

Packaging problems. The Poison Prevention Packaging Act requires that prescription and over-the-counter medications be packaged in childproof containers. In their frustration at attempting to open these containers, patients may break the bottles and either destroy the medication or place it in an unmarked unprotected container. The older person should be made aware that nonchildproof containers are available for prescription medications on request.

Directions for the administration of medications may not be explicit on the packaging, and as a result problems occur. It is assumed that patients know that the foil covering on suppositories must be removed before insertion and that they know how to insert a vaginal or rectal suppository. Package instructions regarding the administration of suppositories, eye and ear drops, eye ointments, and aerosol nasal sprays must be clear and adequately explained to prevent problems of misuse.

Sensorimotor changes. Alterations in hearing, vision, and touch have a profound effect on compliance. Hearing and reading the instructions correctly, seeing the medications clearly, and handling the medications appropriately affect the person's ability to adhere to therapeutic programs. Memory changes that occur may cause a person to forget doses. The person should be informed about what to do if one or more doses are forgotten. Clues to remembering that are discussed in this chapter will improve compliance. Motor changes, especially immobility, may also be a problem in getting the drug from a pharmacy or in self-administration. As an example, administering insulin with hands crippled by arthritis may present a bigger challenge than the patient can manage.

Cost of medication. On an average, the elderly person spends over $100 annually on prescription drugs (Lamy, 1980). This expense is not generally covered by reimbursement plans and presents real problems for persons on limited incomes. A common pattern followed by these persons is to decrease the dose or substitute a less expensive drug that reportedly will have similar results. They should be advised to discuss with the physician the necessity for the drug and the possibility for generic substitution.

Lack of supervision. Older persons living alone or with another person of similar age do not have available to them the direct supervision of a health professional who can answer their questions and make certain that the directions are followed. Family and friends can be instructed with the patient at the time a prescription is filled by the pharmacist or before discharge from a health institution. Referral to a home health service agency for follow-up is advisable when the practitioner suspects that noncompliance may occur.

Assessing compliance

Aware of the problems of noncompliance, the health professional should develop a plan to identify the medication-taking behavior of patients. A variety of mechanisms to assess compliance can be used when patients come to the office, pharmacy, or clinic or when they are seen in their homes. An ideal compliance measurement technique is unobtrusive, objective, practical, and inexpensive. This discussion is limited to mechanisms that meet these criteria.

Assessment mechanisms

Counting dose units. With each visit, patients are instructed to bring their medications with them, at which time the practitioner counts the remaining medications to determine whether the drugs are being taken as prescribed.

Prescription refill patterns. Drugs are generally prescribed for a specified time (e.g., 14 days' supply), and the practitioner can readily determine whether the prescription is being refilled in a regular pattern.

Patient interviews. In an interview, patients may be asked directly how they are taking the medication, and the practitioner can compare their answers with the directions on the container. Another method used in the interviewing process is to ask persons what medications they take each day, beginning in the morning and extending until the following morning. This latter method may be more time consuming, but it is also more effective. Family members can also provide valid information.

Response to therapy. Monitoring the patients' symptoms with each visit will also give an indication of compliance. If they are responding to therapy, an assumption can be made that they are taking the medication correctly. However, the person with a chronic illness such as hypertension may be asymptomatic, a fact that suggests that this mechanism should be used in conjunction with one previously described.

Memory aids for taking medications as directed*

As a means to remember to take medications as directed, several types of memory aids are recommended. Some patients will prefer to devise their own system, and they should be informed that the method selected should help them see at a glance:

Medication to be taken
Amount to be taken
Time to take medication
How to take medication
Whether it has been taken

Four examples of memory aids that can be offered to patients and adapted to their individual needs are included in this chapter. However, patients and practitioners should be reminded that any system is beneficial only if it is carefully used.

SYSTEM I: A CHART OF MEDICATIONS TO BE TAKEN

This simple chart functions as a reminder and provides space for:

Name of drug
Color/shape (or attaching the medication)
Reason for taking
Directions
Times of administration

A completed sample is as follows:

Name of drug	Reason to take	Color and shape	Directions	Time
Digoxin	Regulate pulse	Round, white	One tablet daily	8 AM

SYSTEM II: WEEKLY OR MONTHLY INSTRUCTIONS AND CHECK-OFF CHART

This versatile system can be used as a guide at home with a large calendar or adapted to a smaller format that the patient can carry. Checking off the specific medications ensures that they have been taken at the right time. The system that is presented on p. 62 can be done on a weekly or monthly basis.

*Adapted from Using your medicines wisely: a guide for the elderly, Pub. No. (ADM) 80-75, Washington, D.C., 1979, National Institute on Drug Abuse, U.S. Department of Health, Education, and Welfare.

Name of drug and directions	Sun	Mon	Tue	Wed	Thu	Fri	Sat
Digoxin, one tablet five mornings a week		8	8	8	8	8	
Aspirin, two tablets three times daily with meals	8, 12, 5	8, 12, 5	8, 12, 5	8, 12, 5	8, 12, 5	8, 12, 5	8, 12, 5

SYSTEM III: COLOR CODING

For persons with visual impairment or for persons who prefer this simple method, color coding, which can be done in combination with one of the previously presented systems, may be preferred.

The bottles can be marked with brightly colored adhesive tape or marking pens or a brightly colored tag attached to the bottle. Green and blue are not used since they may be difficult for the older adult to differentiate. Each bottle will be marked in a different color, and the medications on the previously presented charts are marked with the corresponding color. Looking at the chart and the color-coded bottle will help the person select the correct pill and then record that it was taken.

This method is shown in the following:

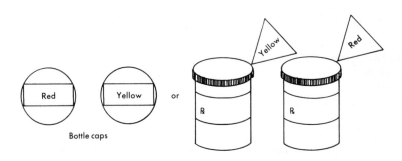

Bottle caps

Name of drug		Sun	Mon	Tue	Wed	Thu	Fri	Sat
Red	Digoxin, one tablet five mornings a week		8	8	8	8	8	
Yellow	Aspirin, two tablets three times daily with meals	8, 12, 5:30	8, 12, 5:30	8, 12, 5:30	8, 12, 5:30	8, 12, 5:30	8, 12, 5:30	8, 12, 5:30

SYSTEM IV: SPECIAL CONTAINERS

A daily container, which may be a cup, pillbox, or other small receptacle, is useful if the person takes only a few pills daily and if it is easy to differentiate the pills by size, shape, or color. The pills are placed in the container each morning, and marking the names of the medicines on the container is advisable. With this method, the person knows at any time of the day how many pills have been taken and how many are left.

For persons who take more pills daily or if the medications look alike, two containers or one larger container is advisable. A morning and afternoon cup may serve this purpose. An egg carton that has 12 cups can be labeled for 12 hours of the day and labeled with the name of the medicine and the dose. The person then will place the medication in the carton cups each day. Commercially available pill counters are also available and can be used in a similar manner.

Factors that interfere with compliance in older persons have been identified, mechanisms to assess medication-taking behavior have been discussed and recommendations that can be made to promote proper taking of medications have been included. Practitioners' taking detailed drug histories using the format presented in Chapter 7 will also help to identify persons not adhering to regimens. They may also learn from patients ingenious methods to help remember to take these medications.

ALCOHOLISM

Alcohol has become one of the most abused drugs in our older population. Alcohol and other drug abuse is defined as intentional, excessive use of substances that are taken to alter the way a person feels. Because of medical advances, alcoholics are living to old age, and an increasing number of older adults are turning to alcohol to ease feelings of depression, loneliness, and loss. Therapy with some older adults has been more successful than with younger populations if the persons and their families can be identified and convinced of therapy. The brief discussion of alcoholism that follows is included because of the noncompliance that may occur as a result of alcohol consumption and because of multiple drug interactions caused by alcohol. Common alcohol-drug interactions are included after the general discussion about alcoholism in older adult populations.

Incidence

The exact incidence of alcoholism in older persons is unclear. However, a record review of alcoholism in this segment of the population (Schuckit and others, 1980) indicates that alcohol problems probably affect between 2% and 10% of the general elderly population, with a higher rate for widowers, persons with medical problems, and persons who are involved with offenses handled by the police. Fairly high rates of alcoholism have been observed in older persons in psychiatric hospitals, mental health clinics, medical-surgical wards of general hospitals, and nursing homes.

Certain groups of older persons are more likely to develop problems associated with alcohol. Vulnerable persons are those encountering the stresses of major life changes: (1) retirement from meaningful work; (2) loss of status and power; (3) alterations in physical and mental health; (4) death of spouse, family, and friends; and (5) change of residence. The health professional should be alert to increased alcohol consumption that may be used to deal with these stresses.

Definition

Alcoholism, although recognized as a disease, is difficult to define because it is not a single disease entity. The National Council of Alcoholism took a step forward in 1972 when it issued a set of criteria to diagnose alcoholism. The criteria have been used to diagnose alcoholic problems more uniformly. Diagnostic clues for the clinical appearance of alcoholism in old age include insomnia, impotence, lack of control of gout, rapid onset of confusional states, uncontrollable hypertension, and unexpected falls (Butler and Lewis, 1982). Alcoholic abuse must be considered as a possible diagnosis in frequent falls, confusion, and self-neglect (Wattis, 1981).

Problems in diagnosing alcoholism

Problems exist in diagnosing alcoholism in the general population, and this situation intensifies in older groups. Families and friends tend to protect the older persons from revealing the situation, and they may deny that drinking is a problem. When the person is thus protected, the drinking increases, alcoholic dependency occurs, and, in a sense, the family is responsible. Family members may also be abusers and are frequently suppliers of alcohol.

Another reason for the problem in diagnosing alcoholism in the older population is the profession's lack of awareness of this health problem. The diagnosis of alcoholism is frequently missed when persons are admitted to health-care facilities. Attention is paid to the medical-physical problems, but the underlying cause may be alcoholism, which is not identified.

In an effort to help a medical staff detect the older patient with alcoholism, Schuckit (1980) offered clues. From his 3-year follow-up study of male alcoholics, he found that this group of men were more likely to live alone and had higher levels of education and occupation than other patients in the same facility. From a medical standpoint, they are more likely to have organic brain syndrome and pulmonary disease. Fortunately, these older alcoholics who seek medical treatment generally stay in for treatment and further care.

Snyder and Way (1979), in their extensive work with older alcoholics, identified some characteristic patterns: alcoholic intake appears to decrease with age, old women drink less than old men, and widowers have the highest incidence and unmarried women the lowest incidence of alcoholism in persons over 69 years of age.

According to the National Council on Alcoholism, the diagnosis of alcoholism is made when one or more of the major criteria of Diagnostic Level I (Criteria for the Diagnosis of Alcoholism) are met. The manifestations as described by these criteria include physical dependency; alcohol-associated illness; tolerance to effects of alcohol; and behavioral, psychological, and attitudinal indexes (drinking despite medical and social contraindications). Screening techniques for the assessment of alcoholic patients, available in the literature (Heinemann and Estes, 1976), are useful as diagnostic tools and aids to planning intervention strategies.

Health problems associated with alcoholism

Multiple and serious pathophysiological changes result from chronic alcohol abuse. Serious changes affect the CNS, gastrointestinal system, cardiovascular system, skeletal system, blood-forming organs, and fluid and electrolyte balance. Malnutrition associated with alcoholism may cause a variety of medical conditions.

Alcohol-drug interactions

The effects of alcohol in combination with drugs are significant for the chronic drinker as well as for the occasional drinker. The Federal Drug Administration Bulletin (June, 1979) focused on the dangers of mixing drugs and alcohol. This study indicated that of the 100 most frequently prescribed drugs, at least half have an ingredient that interacts with alcohol. Alcohol-drug interactions in the general population are responsible for approximately 2500 known deaths and 47,000 emergency department admissions annually. The damage to vital organs caused by chronic alcoholism has a distinct effect on the response of the body to medication, especially when complicated by changes associated with the aging process.

Many responses of the body to alcohol-drug interactions are related to the drug dose as well as to the amount of alcohol consumed. This point emphasizes the need to determine the drinking patterns of older adults while taking a history. Drug doses consequently may be altered and the patient firmly

TABLE 1. Alcohol and drug interactions

Class	Drug	Body response
Analgesics	Aspirin	Gastritis, delayed clotting time, hemorrhage, fecal blood loss.
Antialcohol preparations	Disulfiram	Rise in blood pressure, flushing of face, pounding headache, tachycardia, apprehension, rapid breathing, nausea, vomiting, weakness, dizziness, fainting.
Antianginal and antihypertensive agents	Nitroglycerin, reserpine, methyldopa, hydralazine, guanethidine, peripheral vasodilators	Postural hypotension, fainting, loss of consciousness.
Anticoagulants	Warfarin	Variable according to alcoholic intake and habits; acute intoxication increases anticoagulant effects and hemorrhage; chronic alcoholism decreases anticoagulant effects.
Anticonvulsants	Phenytoin	Increased metabolism of drug causes usual doses to be inadequate.
Antidepressants and stimulants	Tricyclics: desipramine, amitriptyline	Susceptibility to convulsions, hypotension, increased stimulant effect (desipramine), increased depressant effect (amitriptyline).
	MAO inhibitors	Hypertensive crisis when taken with Chianti wine or beer (tyramine-containing beverages).
	Caffeine, amphetamines	Varied behavioral effects.
Antidiabetic agents	Tolbutamide, chlorpropamide, acetohexamide, tolazamide	Unpredictable fluctuations in serum glucose levels, severe hypoglycemia, disulfiram-like reaction.

Adapted from U.S. Department of Health, Education, and Welfare: FDA Drug bulletin **9**(2):2, 1979.

advised of the possible consequences of drinking while taking the prescribed medications. Warnings on the medication container also serve as reminders. The incidence of alcoholism in older persons coupled with the increased sensitivity increases the possibility of alcohol-drug interactions. Table 1 focuses on classes of widely prescribed drugs and their interactions when consumed with alcohol.

TABLE 1. Alcohol and drug interactions—cont'd

Class	Drug	Body response
Antihistamines		Impairment of performance skills, drowsiness.
Antimicrobial/anti-infective agents	Chloramphenicol, griseofulvin, isonia-zid, metronidazole, quinacrine	Nausea, vomiting, headache, possible convulsions.
Barbiturates	Secobarbital, pento-barbital	Drowsiness, impaired motor skills, vomiting, unconsciousness, coma, death.
Major tranquilizers	Chlorpromazine, thioridazine	Hypotension, depressed respiratory function, seizure susceptibility, impaired renal function.
Minor tranquilizers	Meprobamate, benzo-diazepines (fluraze-pam)	Impaired performance skills (driving skills cited), drowsiness.
Narcotics	Hydromorphone, morphine, meperi-dine, propoxyphene	CNS depressant.
Sedative-hypnotics	Chloral hydrate	Tachycardia, palpitations, facial flushing, dysphoria, CNS depressant.

Practitioners' role in increasing the awareness of the dangers of drugs and alcohol

When taking a drug history, the health professional should inquire about the intake of alcohol. Making an inquiry on this sensitive subject may be awkward, but the value has been clearly demonstrated. Asking directly how much alcohol has been consumed over the year, whether that amount has changed, and how much has been consumed in the past week should bring the required information. Validation of this intake may be also done with families. One must bear in mind that the information received may not be true because the patient or family may not want to reveal a drinking problem.

In circumstances in which the hazards of alcohol-drug interactions may occur, older adults should be counseled regarding the adverse effects. A reminder on the medication container and on the accompanying medication instruction sheets, if supplied, will reinforce the teaching. Community education programs for consumers and professionals can also emphasize the hazards of alcohol-drug interactions, the problems of noncompliant behavior that occur in alcoholics, and the effects of alcoholism on the physical/emotional health of older persons. Community resources such as Alcoholics Anonymous, the National Council on Alcoholism, and local mental health associations can be of help to patients, families, and to professionals wishing to make referrals and seek resources to use with patients.

REFERENCES

Butler, R.N., and Lewis, M.I.: Aging and mental health: positive psychosocial approaches, St. Louis, 1982, The C.V. Mosby Co.

Heineman, E., and Estes, N.: Assessing alcoholic patients, Am. J. Nurs. 76:785, 1976.

Lamy, P.: Prescribing for the elderly, Littleton, Mass., 1980, John Wright-PSG, Inc.

Lofholm, P.: Self medication by the elderly. In Kayne, R., editor: Drugs and the elderly, Los Angeles, 1978, University of Southern California Press.

Lundin, D.: Medication taking behavior of the elderly, Drug Intell. Clin. Pharm. 12:518, 1978.

National Council on the Aging: Fact book on aging, Washington, D.C., 1978, the Council.

Schuckit, M., and others: A three year follow-up of alcoholics, J. Clin. Psychiatry 41:412, 1980.

Schwartz, D.: Self medication for elderly patients, Am. J. Nurs. 75:1809, 1975.

Snyder, P., and Way, A.: Alcohol and the elderly, Aging 291-292:8, 1979.

Wattis, J.: Alcoholic problems in the elderly, J. Am. Geriat. Soc. 29:131, 1981.

U.S. Department of Health, Education, and Welfare: FDA Drug Bulletin 9(2):2, 1979.

Using your medicines wisely: a guide for the elderly, Pub. No. (ADM) 80-705, Washington, D.C., 1979, National Institute on Drug Abuse, U.S. Department of Health, Education, and Welfare.

SUGGESTED READINGS

Cheung, A.: Drugs for the aging: use and abuse. In Reinhardt, A.M., and Quinn, M.D., editors: Current practice in gerontological nursing, vol. 1, St. Louis, 1979, The C.V. Mosby Co.

Ebersole, P., and Hess, P.: Toward healthy aging: human needs and nursing response, St. Louis, 1981, The C.V. Mosby Co.

Goldberg, P.B.: How risky is self-care with OTC medicines? Geriatr. Nurs. 1:279, 1980.

Lenhart, D.: The use of medications in the elderly population, Nurs. Clin. North Am. 11:135, 1976.

Schuckit, M.: Geriatric alcoholism and drug abuse, Gerontologist 17:168, 1977.

PROMOTING GOOD NUTRITION IN OLDER ADULTS

6

Good health is promoted by a well-balanced diet through the entire life span. However, the intake of food and essential nutrients in old age is complicated by physical and emotional changes, alterations in life-style, chronic illnesses, and administration of medications. Many drugs that are capable of affecting the nutritional status are used in the treatment of chronic illnesses common among older adults.

This chapter will explore the nutritional needs of older adults; factors that affect the nutritional status, including the influence of medications; guidelines to assessing nutritional status; and recommendations to help promote good nutrition for this group.

NUTRITIONAL NEEDS OF OLDER ADULTS

The nutritional needs of older persons are affected by many factors, including age, body size, metabolism, physical activity, and illness. These variables suggest that the individuality of the person is extremely important in the planning of a dietary program and that the Recommended Dietary Allowances of the National Academy of Sciences serve as general guidelines from which individual programs are planned.

Calories

With increasing age, a gradual reduction in energy takes place. Lowered metabolic rates, decrease in physical activities, decrease in total body cells, and decrease in lean body mass are factors that indicate the need to reduce caloric intake as people grow older. The Food and Nutrition Board of the National Academy of Sciences has recommended that caloric allowances be decreased by 5% between ages 22 and 35, by 3% each decade between ages 35 and 55, by 5% each decade between ages 55 and 75, and by an additional 7% after age 75. These guidelines offer a general perspective of lowered calorie requirements for older adults, but they do not specify exact requirements.

Caloric needs will vary with each person because of the variations in physical activity patterns, amount of rest, and overall metabolic needs. A general guide to requirements is the observation of the person's weight gain and loss on a particular diet. Consuming more calories than needed will lead to the retention of calories in the form of excess fat, which is detrimental to general body functioning. The incidence of obesity peaks in the forties for women and the sixties for men. Generally lower body weights occur in the population over 60 years of age. This decrease reflects changes in food intake and also the change in the composition of the groups who are generally in better physical condition.

Weg (1978) argues that a diet with decreased calories may deprive a person of essential nutrients. She emphasizes the need for individuality in planning diets for all persons. The low-calorie diets, which include many of the fad diets, may be deficient in fats and carbohydrates, which are the principal fuels for energy. If these fuels are deficient, the body, using protein for fuel, depletes itself of protein needed for tissue repair and maintenance.

Regular measurements of weight are essential in assessing caloric intake. However, weight changes in older persons may result from changes in body composition caused by chronic illness, such as edema, not necessarily from caloric intake.

Protein

Protein and the essential amino acids are required by the body for the synthesis of protein and other nitrogen-containing substances. The need for protein remains fairly constant throughout life, and despite conflicting evidence, there is little reason to believe that the need decreases with age. Healthy older adults who are generally able to use protein effectively require 0.8 gm/kg of body weight, but that amount needs to be increased during infection, illness, disease, and psychological stress.

Dietary protein is derived from several sources that are generally classed as meat and vegetable. Animal sources, which are complete proteins, are derived from meat, poultry, fish, milk, cheese, and eggs. Vegetable proteins, which are also essential to a person's daily diet, are derived from plant products such as dried beans, rice, wheat, corn, and other grains. Because plant sources of protein may not contain all the essential amino acids, combinations of vegetables are necessary for persons on diets limited to vegetable proteins. Older persons should be encouraged to eat high-quality protein from animal sources and to supplement the diet with less expensive vegetable proteins. Personal preferences that are based on culture and economic status and the ability to chew need to be considered by the practitioner recommending protein foods.

Carbohydrates

Meeting the carbohydrate requirements in an older population is not a matter of grave concern, except for the quality of the nutrient. Older persons may consume large amounts of refined carbohydrates because they are inexpensive and immediately satisfying. Complex carbohydrates (the starches) found in the nutrient-rich grains and beans and the natural simple sugars found in fruits and vegetables are desirable sources of this nutrient. Increasing the consumption of these foods provides a good source of essential vitamins, minerals, and trace nutrients, as well as fiber. Attention has been drawn to the fiber in our diet. Epidemiological studies (Burkitt and Meisner, 1979) have shown that diverticulosis, colon cancer, hiatal hernias, and hemorrhoids are less prevalent in parts of the world where fiber consumption is high. The most important function of fiber is to bind water in the intestine in the form of a gel. This prevents its overabsorption from the large bowel and ensures that the fecal content of the large bowel is bulky and smooth, a consistency that allows easy passage.

The best sources of fiber are foods with a lower water content. Root vegetables (potatoes, parsnips, and carrots), legumes (peas, beans, and millet), minimally processed cereals (bran), and whole-grain breads are good sources. Fruits and leafy vegetables should be eaten for vitamin content, but their fiber content is lower.

Fat

The diet of the typical person living in this country is high in fat, with an estimated 40% to 45% of the daily intake of calories taken from this source. Fats are a necessary component of the diet because they serve as a vehicle for the fat-soluble vitamins A, D, E, and K. They also enhance the flavor of food, give the person a feeling of fullness, and reduce the amount of acid secretion and muscular activity of the stomach.

The fat in the American diet is derived primarily from animal sources, but the trend is toward increasing vegetable sources, especially the unsaturated fats. The continuing controversy surrounding the role of fats in elevated serum cholesterol and the relationship of increased serum cholesterol to the development of atherosclerosis has increased public awareness of the value of including unsaturated fats in the diet. Cholesterol levels continue to rise as people grow older, which may be related to food intake, aging, and other factors.

Nutritionists recommend reduction in fats, particularly cholesterol and saturated fats, for persons whose cholesterol levels are above the 50th percentile for the older age group. Practitioners should recognize the need for individuality in this recommendation. A person of 80 who eats a high-fat diet and is in reasonably good health may not be a candidate for this change, but a younger person with cholesteremia may be a candidate for a diet lower in total fats with an increase in polyunsaturated fats.

Vitamins

The need for each of the vitamins remains essentially the same throughout adult life. These nutrients, which are found in a wide variety of food, function as catalysts in the chemical reactions that support the body's physiological functions. However, the elderly are susceptible to vitamin deficiencies because their diets may have inadequate quantities of food from natural sources, particularly fruits and vegetables.

Vague symptoms of weakness and fatigue, often attributed to old age, may result from prolonged inadequate vitamin intake. When old age is complicated with chronic illness, additional vague complaints of suboptimum performance, decreased resistance to infection, and slow wound healing may be responsive to vitamin-mineral supplementation.

Many misconceptions exist about the need for supplemental vitamins in the American diet. Advertising has been effective in selling the supplements by promising improved health, vigor, and energy. Unfortunately, there have been few well-controlled studies on the effects of vitamin supplementation. Studies have indicated deficiencies of vitamins A and C, but when consumers select vitamins, they are unaware of the vitamins they need and will select a multiple vitamin. They also fall victim to the highly advertised claims for megadoses of vitamins, failing to understand the possible adverse effects of some of these nutrients. The fat-soluble vitamins A and D and more recently E and K are known to have toxic effects in large amounts. Of the water-soluble vitamins, C, niacin, B_6 (pyridoxine), and folic acid also have adverse effects when taken in large doses.

Vitamins from natural sources are recommended, and if a deficiency is diagnosed through the identification of specific symptoms, the health professional can recommend supplemental vitamins.

Minerals

As with vitamins, the need for minerals remains fairly constant through-out adult life. The minerals are well distributed in food, except for calcium and iron. Older adults frequently have deficiencies in these two nutrients, and these deficiencies lead to health problems involving the hemopoietic and skeletal systems. Special attention will be given to these nutrients, which when taken in required amounts through natural sources and supplements can prevent debilitating health problems.

Calcium

When calcium is deficient in the diet over an extended period, demin-eralization of the bones increases. Calcium is necessary to maintain the normal bone matrix. As persons grow older, negative calcium balance exists, more calcium is lost, and osteoporosis occurs. Other factors that contribute to calcium deficiency include impaired absorption of calcium, deficiency of vitamin D, and decreased physical activity that may promote increased ex-cretion of calcium.

Reversing the process of calcium loss is not accomplished by simply con-suming more of this mineral. Vitamin D is necessary to stimulate intestinal absorption of calcium and phosphate, decrease renal absorption, and en-hance resorption of bone. Authorities agree that increasing the calcium in-take to 1 to 1.5 gm daily will help to restore calcium balance. However, it is doubtful that the calcium will prevent or arrest the development of osteo-porosis.

Iron

Older persons may be vulnerable to the problems associated with iron deficiency because of lack of knowledge of iron-rich foods, poor dietary habits, and lack of financial resources to purchase good natural sources of iron. Chronic blood loss, poor absorption, and inadequate use of iron are also factors in the development of iron-deficiency anemia. Increased incidence of anemia has been found among poor elderly, but anemia is not necessarily part of the aging process.

Good dietary sources of iron include fish and meat. Eggs, spinach, and a few other vegetables contain high iron content, but since they form insoluble salts, the amount of iron available for absorption is decreased.

Water

Water is not generally considered food, but an adequate supply of fluid is essential for normal body functioning. It provides the environment in which all chemical reactions take place, is vital for urinary excretion mechanisms, helps prevent constipation, and acts as an expectorant to liquify respiratory excretions. Sufficient fluid should be consumed daily to provide a 24-hour output of 1000 to 1500 ml of urine. Thirst will usually stimulate fluid intake, but the thirst mechanism in older persons may lose this regulatory function. They may need assistance in establishing a plan of fluid intake that will adequately hydrate the body. Withholding fluids late in the day as a means of preventing nocturia should be discouraged, because dehydration can occur within a short time.

FACTORS AFFECTING THE NUTRITIONAL STATUS OF OLDER ADULTS

The older population is affected by many factors that influence their nutritional status, which is determined by the intake of food and the use of the nutrients.

Intake of food

The life changes encountered by older persons greatly influence patterns of food intake. The reduction of income that is imposed by retirement limits the variety of foods available for purchase, a limitation that in turn affects the availability of nutrients required in a well-balanced diet, particularly fresh fruits and vegetables. The decrease in income may also necessitate a change in living arrangements, depriving persons of food storage areas in their homes. Cooking and refrigeration units may differ, and this difference requires an adaptation to change that may become more difficult as persons grow older. With the loss of working colleagues, family, and friends through illness or death, the circle of relationships grows smaller, and the incidence of depression increases as persons are unable to reach out to others. Associated with the multiple loss is the lack of appetite, which has a marked effect on proper intake of food.

Physical changes have a definite effect on proper intake of food. The ability to smell and taste the food declines with aging. The loss of this ability influences the perception of the flavor of food, which no longer has the appeal that it had when the person was younger. The decline in the number and size of taste buds on the tongue, loss of teeth, ill-fitting dentures, decrease in salivary flow, and changes in the oral mucosa greatly affect the type of food eaten, which often becomes monotonous and uninspiring. Mealtime ceases to be the pleasure of previous years.

Many older adults are required to limit their sodium intake because of medical conditions such as hypertension and congestive heart failure and also because of medications such as diuretics and digitalis. It is a common misconception that omitting salt at the table constitutes a low-sodium diet. Most people are unaware of the sodium that occurs naturally in some foods and the sodium that is added in processing. Processed foods are frequently relied on because they are more convenient to purchase, are designed for one or two persons, and are easier to prepare. A simple example will illustrate the sodium added in processing. Three fourths cup of regular oatmeal cooked in unsalted water contains 1 mg of sodium, but the same amount of instant oatmeal contains 250 mg of sodium. Offering patients lists of foods high in sodium will help them to plan menus that will maximize effects of medications and generally promote health.

Perceptual changes in vision and hearing may affect patterns of intake of nutrients. Visual changes such as presbyopia, the decreased ability to adapt to darkness, and the need for increased illumination make it difficult for older adults to enjoy a meal in a restaurant with dim lighting. Auditory changes, characterized by an inability to distinguish high-frequency sounds, may make older persons reluctant to eat in public places or at social gatherings because they feel isolated when they cannot enjoy the conversation.

Handicaps associated with chronic illnesses, such as the residual paralysis following a stroke and the weakness associated with heart disease, can interfere with shopping for, preparing, and eating food. These illnesses may require that the diet be altered to eliminate some of the favorite foods, and this elimination can affect the joys previously associated with eating.

Use of food

Digestion and the ultimate use of food are affected by a variety of phenomena associated with aging or pathological changes. Among the important changes are degeneration of the salivary glands, which is accompanied by a loss of digestive enzymes; decreased production and delivery of enzymes of the stomach, pancreas, and small intestines; and changes in bile released by the gallbladder and liver. There are also structural changes that affect the quantity of enzymes that are excreted, stored, and used. The vascular system no longer delivers the amount of blood that once nourished the gastrointestinal organs, and this change eventually affects the use of vital nutrients.

Influence of drugs
Drug-induced nutrient deficiencies

Drug-induced vitamin deficiencies (Table 2) have become increasingly more significant as more drugs are available and polypharmacy becomes more common among older persons. Some drugs may impair the appetite, and this impairment reduces the intake of nutrients. Other drugs may affect

TABLE 2. Drug-induced vitamin deficiencies

Vitamin	Drug	Results of deficiencies
A	Mineral oil Neomycin	Xerophthalmia Night blindness Keratinization of epithelium Skin and mucous membrane infections
B_1	Antacids Antibacterial agents	Gastrointestinal system: anorexia, gastric atony, indigestion, deficiency of hydrochloric acid CNS: fatigue, apathy, neuritis, paralysis Cardiovascular system: cardiac failure, peripheral vascular dilatation, edema of extremities
B_2	Cathartics Neomycin	Poor wound healing Cracks at corners of mouth (cheilosis) Glossitis Eye irritation and photophobia Seborrheic dermatitis
B_6	Isoniazid Hydralazine Cycloserine Neomycin	Anemia CNS: hyperirritability, convulsions, neuritis
B_{12}	Trifluoperazine Colchicine	Pernicious anemia
C	Tobacco products (smoking)	Delayed wound healing
D	Photosensitizing drugs Mineral oil	Rickets Faulty bone growth Osteomalacia
K	Antibacterial agents Mineral oil	Unusual bruising or bleeding
Folic acid	Phenytoin Primidone Barbiturates Methotrexate Trimethoprim	Anemia (megaloblastic)

absorption, increase renal excretion, or interfere with metabolism and use. Roe (1976) has identified factors that increase the risk of drug-induced vitamin deficiencies:

Pharmacological properties of the drug
Prolonged drug use or abuse
Slow rate of drug absorption
Inadequate vitamin intake
Extent of physical change of aging
Disease process
Concurrent alcohol abuse

Other factors that may be responsible for drug-induced deficiencies include drugs that cause depression, anorexia, nausea, and gastric irritation or alter taste sensation.

Drugs that interfere with nutrient absorption and use have been categorized into eight major drug groups (Fitzgerald, 1980):

1. Drugs affecting gastric or intestinal motility—mineral oil, for example, decreases the absorption of carotenes and vitamins A, D, E, and K; bisacodyl, phenolphthalein, and other laxatives decrease intestinal uptake of glucose; excessive use of antacids can result in thiamine (vitamin B_1) deficiency.

2. Drugs used to reduce cholesterol—clofibrate and cholestyramine have been associated with malabsorption of vitamin B_{12}, iron, electrolytes, and sugar.

3. Surface-active agents—stool softeners can have effects on fat dispersion and permeability of lipoprotein membranes that result in changes in absorption of several nutrients.

4. Antiinfective agents—neomycin, erythromycin, tetracyclines, penicillins, chloramphenicol, sulfonamides, isoniazid, and others have been implicated in decreased use of folic acid, malabsorption of vitamin B_{12}, decreased bacterial synthesis of vitamin K, and impaired absorption of calcium and magnesium.

5. Cytotoxic drugs—methotrexate antagonizes folic acid and interferes with the absorption of vitamin B_{12}. Colchicine, used in the treatment of acute gout, is associated with malabsorption of vitamin B_{12}, carotene, fat, lactose, and electrolytes.

6. Anticonvulsant drugs—phenytoin and phenobarbital interfere with the use of folic acid and vitamins B_{12} and D.

7. Diuretics—most diuretics, except triamterene and spironolactone, can precipitate hypokalemia by excessive potassium loss.

8. Alcohol—alcohol can cause malabsorption of folic acid and vitamin B_{12} and increased excretion of magnesium.

Drugs causing gastric irritation

Drugs causing gastric irritation may depress the appetite; cause abdominal bloating, fullness, or pain; or result in nausea and vomiting. Medications prescribed for older persons that may cause these side effects include aminophylline, aspirin, chlorpromazine, ferrous salts, hydrochlorothiazide, hydrocortisone, indomethacin, isoniazid, potassium salts, prednisone, reserpine, tolbutamide, triamterene, trihexyphenidyl, and trimeprazine.

ASSESSING THE NUTRITIONAL STATUS OF OLDER ADULTS

Determining the presence of nutritional problems in older persons is a significant component of any evaluation. Practitioners in various health fields are aware of the need for nutritional well-being, and the suggestions that follow may be adapted to various professions and situations.

The cornerstone of a nutritional assessment is the dietary history. Taking and recording this history is time consuming and requires much patience, and in some circumstances the history may not be accurate. Several approaches can be used in obtaining the essential information. A good screening tool that has proved to be fairly reliable is to offer persons lists of foods in major categories and have them indicate the number of times per week these foods are eaten. This method helps to identify persons who follow fad diets, who eat almost exclusively from one or two categories of food, who consume large amounts of empty calories, and who have unusual dietary problems that may exclude certain foods or food groups.

A more traditional method of obtaining a dietary history includes asking the person about all foods and liquids consumed in the past 24 hours. Recall beyond that span of time is frequently unreliable because of changes in recent memory and because of erratic meals. With careful instruction, the patient or family member can keep a record of food and fluid intake for a 3-day period, which offers a good nutritional picture. Practitioners should recognize that keeping a record has a positive effect on dietary intake.

Other essential information the practitioner should inquire about includes eating habits, distribution of meals, omission of meals, type and frequency of snacks, and nutritional supplements. The history may also be more valuable if the practitioner inquires about who purchases and prepares the food, facilities for storing food, whether the person eats alone or with someone, and whether food has special significance.

A drug history may also reveal nutritional problems related to medications. Drugs may be causing nausea and gastric irritation affecting food intake, or they may be affecting the absorption and use of nutrients. Conversely, foods may be affecting the absorption and use of medications.

GUIDELINES IN PROMOTING GOOD NUTRITION

Health practitioners can help promote good nutrition in older persons by:
- Informing patients of the components of a well-balanced diet and giving examples of foods that achieve that balance
- Encouraging a wide variety of foods to stimulate the appetite and provide varied nutrients
- Suggesting foods that are good sources of vitamins A and C, calcium, and iron, which are often deficient in the diets of older persons
- Encouraging the ingestion of high-fiber foods, fresh fruits and vegetables, and grains to promote regular bowel habits
- Recommending drinking 6 to 8 full glasses of water daily to encourage good general body functioning
- Promoting regular exercise that will stimulate the appetite, aid digestion, and burn up extra calories
- Discussing with patients the effects of medications on nutritional status
- Advising patients of vitamin and mineral deficiencies that may occur with specific medications and suggesting foods rich in nutrients that will correct these deficiencies
- Referring patients to community nutrition programs that serve a well-balanced diet at low cost
- Referring persons with suspected nutritional deficiencies to a qualified nutritionist

Following this section are a variety of charts and tables that can be used as resources in counseling older adults about good nutrition (Table 3 and the boxes below and on pp. 80-82).

FOODS HIGH IN POTASSIUM

Apricots	Kidney beans	Pineapple
Avocados	Lentils	Pork
Bananas	Liver	Prunes
Beef	Mushrooms	Raisins
Beets	Nonfat milk	Sardines
Chicken	Nuts	Soybeans
Dates	Onions	Tangerines
Dried milk	Orange juice	Tomato juice
Figs (dried)	Peaches	Tomato puree
Fish (fresh)	Peas	Veal

FOODS HIGH IN SODIUM

Salted meats (such as ham and bacon)
Sausages
Canned vegetables and soups
Dairy products
Chinese foods
Commercially baked breads and biscuits
Ready-to-eat breakfast cereals
Frozen plate dinners
Snacks (such as pretzels and chips)
Salad dressing
Condiments (such as mustard, catsup, and soy sauce)

TABLE 3. Recommended dietary allowances for persons over 51 years of age designed for maintenance of good nutrition of practically all healthy people in the United States

Vitamin/mineral	Weight	Males*	Females*
Protein	g	56	44
Vitamin A	μg	1000	800
Vitamin D	μg	5	5
Vitamin E	mg	10	8
Vitamin C	mg	60	60
Thiamine	mg	1.2	1.0
Riboflavin	mg	1.4	1.2
Niacin	mg	16	13
Vitamin B_6	mg	2.2	2.0
Folic acid	μg	400	400
Vitamin B_{12}	μg	3.0	3.0
Calcium	mg	800	800
Phosphorus	mg	800	800
Magnesium	mg	350	300
Iron	mg	10	10
Zinc	mg	15	15
Iodine	μg	150	150

Adapted from information from the Food and Nutrition Board, National Academy of Sciences, National Research Council, Washington, D.C., 1980.
*Requirements for males 70 inches tall, 154 pounds; females 64 inches tall, 120 pounds.

FOOD GUIDE FOR OLDER ADULTS (MINIMUM REQUIREMENTS)

MILK GROUP—2 SERVINGS DAILY

Nutrients	Leading source of calcium and riboflavin; excellent source of protein and vitamin A.
Types of food	Milk (whole, skim, evaporated, powdered, buttermilk), yogurt, cheese, ice cream.
Suggestions	With restricted calories or fat, skim milk and low-fat yogurt are good sources; 8 ounces of milk or yogurt has the same amount of calcium as 1½ slices of cheddar cheese, 1¾ cups of ice cream, or 2 cups of cottage cheese.

FRUIT-VEGETABLE GROUP—4 SERVINGS DAILY

Nutrients	Leading source of vitamins A and C.
Types of food	Citrus fruits, dark green leafy or orange vegetables.
Suggestions	1 serving of citrus fruit daily for vitamin C; 3-4 servings of dark green or orange vegetables per week. One adult serving is 1 cup raw fruit or vegetable, ½ cup cooked fruit or vegetable, 1 medium fruit (apple or banana), or ½ cup fruit juice.

MEAT GROUP—2 SERVINGS DAILY

Nutrients	Protein, niacin, thiamine, riboflavin, iron.
Types of food	Meat, poultry, fish, eggs, dried beans, or peas.
Suggestions	1 serving of meat, fish, or poultry daily. 3-4 eggs weekly if there are no cholesterol restrictions. One adult serving is 2 ounces of meat, fish, or poultry, 2 eggs, 1 cup cooked dried beans, peas, or lentils; or 4 tablespoons peanut butter.

GRAIN GROUP—4 SERVINGS DAILY

Nutrients	Carbohydrate, thiamine, riboflavin, niacin, iron.
Types of food	Whole-grain, fortified, or enriched grain products are recommended; this group includes bread, cereals, noodles, macaroni, and other pasta.
Suggestions	One adult serving is 1 slice bread; 1 cup ready-to-eat cereal; ½ cup cooked cereal, pasta, cornmeal, rice, or grits; 1 small muffin or biscuit; or 2 graham crackers.

SOURCES OF PRINCIPAL VITAMINS

FAT SOLUBLE	SOURCE
A	Butter, fortified margarine, liver, carrots, sweet potatoes, yams, tomatoes, leafy greens, broccoli, cantaloupe, winter squash, apricots, peaches, juices of these fruits and vegetables
D	Fortified milk, fortified margarine, fish liver oils
E	Vegetable oils, wheat germ, milk, eggs, fish, beef, pork, poultry
K	Green leafy vegetables

WATER SOLUBLE	SOURCE
C (ascorbic acid)	Oranges, grapefruit, lemons, strawberries, tangerines, cantaloupe, honeydew melon, watermelon, broccoli, cabbage, cauliflower, green peppers, asparagus, brussels sprouts, potatoes, sweet potatoes, tomatoes, turnips, leafy greens, juices of these foods
B_1 (thiamine)	Pork, beef liver, nuts, dried beans, peas, whole-grain or enriched breads and cereal, enriched or brown rice, enriched pasta, noodles and other flour products, potatoes
B_2 (riboflavin)	Milk, enriched and whole grain products, meat, fish, poultry, eggs, liver, cheese
B_3 (niacin)	Beef, poultry, pork, liver, beans, peas, peanuts, potatoes, enriched grain products
B_6 (pyridoxine)	Found in small amounts in many foods; best sources: beef, poultry, pork, organ meats, wheat and corn products, soybeans, lima beans, yeast
B_{12} (cobalamin)	Beef; poultry; pork; organ meats; shellfish; tongue; fish; milk; eggs; cheese; dried, cooked, or canned peas, beans, lentils, tofu, nuts
Folate (folic acid)	Dried beans and nuts, leafy green vegetables, organ meats, whole grains, yeast

REFERENCES

Burkitt, D , and Meisner, P.: How to manage constipation with high-fiber diet, Geriatrics **34:**33, 1979.
Fitzgerald, W.: Food-drug interactions, Professional Practice Newsletter of American College of Apothecaries **5**(1):1, 1980.
Roe, D.: Drug induced nutritional deficiencies, Westport, Conn., 1976, AVI Publishing Co.
Weg, R.: Nutrition and the later years, Los Angeles, 1978, University of Southern California Press.

SUGGESTED READINGS

Albanese, A.: Calcium nutrition in the elderly, Postgrad. Med. **63:**176, 1978.
Bozian, M.: Nutrition for the aged or aged nutrition? Nurs. Clin. North Am. **11:**169, 1976.
Kutchevesky, D.: How aging affects cholesterol metabolism, Postgrad. Med. **63:**133, 1978.
Munro, H.: Major gaps in nutrient allowances, J. Am. Diet. Assoc. **76:**137, 1980.
Schlesinger, D., and others.: Food patterns in an urban population: age and demographic correlates, J. Gerontol. **35:**432, 1980.
Todhunter, E.N., and Darby, W.J.: Guidelines for maintaining adequate nutrition in old age, Geriatrics **33:**49, 1978.
Virginia Council on Health and Medical Care: Nutrition education for the elderly, Richmond, 1978, Virginia Council on Health and Medical Care.
Williams, E.J.: Food for thought: meeting the nutrition needs of the elderly, Nursing **10:**61, 1980.

7

TEACHING THE OLDER ADULT

Older people can continue to learn from practitioners who have developed a philosophy of education that is geared to them. If health-care workers believe that patient education is an essential component of care, they will develop basic skills and provide opportunities for patients to learn to adapt to the life adjustments related to aging. Nurses and pharmacists are in a unique position to help older persons assume more responsibility in the management of their health-illness conditions. Both professions, by contributing to the educational process, can enable the older person to become more independent and to maintain an optimum level of health.

Health education is the process that bridges the gap between health information and health practices. As health educators, nurses and pharmacists can help bridge that gap by developing individual and group programs in areas such as medication, diet, and exercise. A basic tenet of those who believe in practitioner involvement in patient education is that greater knowledge improves patient compliance and thereby improves patient outcomes. Problems of noncompliance that were identified in a previous chapter form the rationale for teaching older persons about their medications and their correct administration.

FACTORS AFFECTING THE LEARNING PROCESS

Multiple changes that affect the ability to learn occur in the older person's body. Alterations in vision and hearing, variations in intelligence, changes in memory and problem-solving ability, education, socioeconomic status, and overall health status have an effect on the learning process. Each of these factors will be explored.

Vision

Over time certain changes that occur in the structure and function of the eye can affect the ability of the older person to learn as well as take medication accurately. The lens, which must be able to change shape to focus on near and far objects, undergoes alteration. As a person ages, cellular growth slows and a progressive accumulation of old tissue occurs at the center of the lens, making the lens less transparent, yellowish, and rigid. This change results in lack of flexibility, which makes it more difficult for the ciliary muscle to change the shape of the lens, a slow and less complete ability to accommodate to near and far vision, and a decreased ability to discriminate colors in the blue, blue-green, and violet range.

Changes in the iris result in an increased need for light and the loss of speed in accommodating to changes in light and dark. Since the narrowed pupil also affects the amount of light that enters the eye, it becomes necessary to increase the amount of lighting to promote safety and comfort. The eye of a 60-year-old person requires twice the illumination of that of a 20-year-old for a given task. The ciliary muscles also become less elastic and as a result are less functional.

This change in the ciliary muscle, combined with the decreased compliance of the lens, contributes to problems of accommodating to distance. Because the eye brings visual changes to focus on the retina by changing the shape and refractive power of the lens, near vision requires an increased amount of work by the ciliary muscle. However, when the muscle has lost some of its ability to contract, near vision is compromised, and corrective lenses are then essential for close work.

Eye changes require that the health practitioner carefully assess the visual ability of the individual older adult and use this assessment to determine the need for more light and large print teaching tools. If glasses are necessary, they must be accessible, clean, and properly fitted. In situations in which color discrimination is necessary, such as urine tests, it may not be possible for the patient to interpret the results. A careful assessment of visual status is essential when the practitioner is assisting the patient in promotion of self-care.

The following suggestions will guide the practitioner when teaching the older adult with visual impairment:

Provide adequate lighting at all times.

Avoid glare of sunlight and glossy surfaces.

Keep eyeglasses clean and convenient.

Use large print materials.

Use contrasting colors for resources; do not use blue, green, or purple.

Hearing

Subtle changes in hearing begin to occur in persons in their midforties, with a progressive loss as aging continues. Population studies indicate that approximately half the population over 65 has some hearing deficit, and by 80 years of age, 65% have serious hearing problems. Hearing impairment can have a profound effect on the health professional's attempts to teach the person about medications and other health measures.

Major problems in hearing in older adults are loss of auditory acuity, increased sensitivity to loud and extraneous sounds, distortion of sounds, and reduced speed in auditory processing. These difficulties result in problems of auditory discrimination. The older adult has particular difficulty hearing high tones. Consonants (t, s, sh, f, v) that are examples of high tones are particularly difficult for the older person to discriminate. In addition to the high tone, the consonant is of short duration and low power, and use of them may result in distorted perception. Understanding portions of words becomes increasingly difficult when words are complex and rapidly spoken, and there is excessive background noise.

The health professional should be aware of other signs of hearing loss, as evidenced by cupping the hand to the ear, leaning forward, watching the speaker's face intently, and giving inappropriate responses. Family members may also report behaviors such as social withdrawal, depression, paranoia, inattentiveness, and inappropriate responses, which may indicate hearing impairment.

The following suggestions will guide the practitioner in communicating with the older adult who has a hearing impairment:

Face the person when speaking.

Maintain eye contact.

Direct the voice to the ear that has the best hearing.

Keep your mouth visible, since the person may read lips.

Allow the light to fall on the speaker's face.

Enunciate words clearly.

Speak at a moderate pace with normal articulation.

Speak in a normal to lower tone of voice.

Do not shout, because it raises the tone of the voice.

Change to a new subject at a slower rate, offering clues to the change.

Frame questions in different words if responses are inappropriate.

Use multiple visual cues.

Reduce background noise.

Allow the person ample time to respond.

Intelligence

When the cognitive processes are considered, the assumption is made that the decline of intelligence is inevitable. However, evidence in this area is conflicting. The use of traditional tests of intelligence has been attacked because the tests were designed to measure the skills of white, middle-class children and young adults. When intelligence tests consist of items related to the needs of adults, the scores tend to rise during the middle and later years. Tests that emphasize verbal skills show minimal if any decline, whereas those that emphasize psychomotor performance show a greater decline.

When the significance of intelligence in older populations is considered, a differentiation must be made between fluid and crystallized intelligence. Crystallized abilities, which are a function of information, skills, and experience, are transmitted to the individual by the culture and do not diminish. Fluid abilities, or speed and reaction time, do diminish and probably are a result of biological age changes. Knowledge of these factors should be considered in teaching.

Multiple factors that can affect intelligence in the older adult are personality characteristics, motivation, socioeconomic status, education, experience, and physical and mental health. In planning learning opportunities the practitioner should be aware that intellectual functioning remains stable until shortly before death.

Memory and learning

Age-related memory losses have been widely reported in the literature, but the rate of loss occurring with advancing age is highly individual, both in rate and decline. Bright people and persons who exercise their memories reportedly are less susceptible to memory loss.

Memory is an organized network of concepts and ideas that are interrelated in specific ways. If the interrelationships among these concepts are not used because of loss, decreased retrieval, or slower access, the person loses the spontaneous use of memory links, and memory deficits become apparent.

Short-term memory shows the greatest evidence of loss in the older person. Since the short-term memory is susceptible to interferences from other activities, it is difficult for the person to focus on remembering. The amount of new information the person receives probably affects the ability to remember the details of the new concepts being learned.

The health professional who is teaching the older person should attempt to control the number of distractions and disruptions in the learning environment. Presenting limited information at one time will enhance the ability to recall. If the setting is quiet and activity is limited, the person is better able to direct attention to the task at hand. Offering the person an opportunity to recall information immediately following its presentation and a week or two later will improve the ability to remember.

Reaction time, which is traditionally defined as the period between stimulation and initiation of a response, increases with age. The increase is very slight for simple tasks but becomes greater as the tasks get more complex. The more choices involved in the task, the longer the person takes to react. When the stimulus duration is long, older adults react more slowly. Two factors may relate to this slower reaction: (1) inefficiency in initiating the response and (2) caution in initiating the response. The older person spends more time checking responses when in the testing situation. The extent of slowing differs widely from task to task.

Caution that increases with the aging process can result from discomfort with uncertainty and the fear of failure. The older person seeks certainty before being willing to make a response. The hesitation in responding can therefore be viewed as a precautionary measure. Risk taking is not a characteristic aging behavior. Allowing an adequate amount of information and sufficient amount of time to respond will help to decrease this cautious behavior.

The reaction time in learning is complicated by the nature of the stimulus, complexity and type of response required, amount of extraneous information, and the rate of presentation. Since the older person requires more time to process information than does a younger person, material must be presented at a slower pace to facilitate learning. Self-paced learning with appropriate feedback, which allows more time for learning in a relaxed environment, will improve the learning process.

Problem solving

Problem solving is the development of decisions out of processes of reason, logic, and thought. In this process, the older person is at a disadvantage because many items must be dealt with simultaneously. There is difficulty in attaching meaning to stimuli and later remembering this information when attempting to arrive at a solution. The older adult generally does not proceed in an orderly style, has trouble eliminating irrelevant data, and is overwhelmed by multiple facts. As a result, the number of errors rises with age in problem-solving situations. Alternative teaching methods should be used if this occurs.

Health-illness status

The health-illness status of an older adult greatly affects the ability to learn because of the energies directed toward healing and maintenance of health. The loss of the ability to concentrate, which greatly affects a person's learning skills, often accompanies physical or mental illness. Because 80%

of persons who are over 65 have one or more chronic illnesses, the health worker can suspect that there may be an effect on learning; therefore a careful evaluation is necessary.

Socioeconomic status

The lifelong socioeconomic status has implications for the older adult learner. The commitment to mastery of new knowledge and the learning style are two factors that are affected. Persons of higher socioeconomic status tend to seek information from mass media and experts, whereas blue-collar workers seek new information from informal, interpersonal contact with family and friends. Knowledge of this information-seeking behavior can be used in planning teaching strategies for this population.

Educational level

The ability to learn also depends on a person's level of formal education. Many persons over 65 years of age never had the opportunity to attend high school, and college education was uncommon when they were young. The lack of formal education does not mean the person cannot learn, but the health professional must carefully assess the level of formal and informal education to plan a desirable teaching program.

STRATEGIES FOR TEACHING OLDER ADULTS
Thorough assessment precedes the program planning process

Because of the heterogeneity of the older adult population, a thorough assessment must be done by the health professional. The baseline data drawn from this process will provide the nurse, pharmacist, or other health practitioner with essential information that can have a profound effect on the learning process. The assessment can also have a positive effect on the nurse-patient or pharmacist-patient relationship, which in turn can affect the patient's receptivity to learning.

Physical comfort based on needs is provided

All learners require physical comfort, but the changes accompanying the aging process create a special need. Factors such as sensory deficits and arthritic changes demand that the room arrangement be mobile and chairs be adaptable. The room should be well lighted, have minimal distractions, and be located near rest rooms. Room temperature should be adjusted to promote comfort, and breaks should be scheduled to allow the person time to relax and absorb information.

Involving patients in planning enhances the learning process

The practitioner needs to work with the patient to establish meaningful short- and long-term goals. Agreeing on these goals and how they can best be achieved helps the practitioner focus on the essential content and method. The patient can also help select the type of medium that will be most helpful in learning. Conferring about the most effective learning method, for example, visual or auditory, can provide valuable information regarding media selection.

Older persons are encouraged to participate in as many decisions as possible

Older adults are capable of making many decisions, since they have had many such opportunities. Their lives have been rich with such experiences, and they are ingenious in reaching good decisions. Allowing them to decide when, how, and what learning will occur will enhance the learning process. They may not have adequate information to make a decision, but the practitioner can provide the information and tools to make a decision. However, in situations such as dependency, older persons may need more help or someone to make a decision for them.

Participative learning gets adults actively involved in the learning process

Participative learning is an effective teaching method that can be used with older adults. Experiential techniques and simulation exercises are effective in facilitating adult learning. Demonstrations and return demonstrations, perhaps of a particular treatment, such as administering insulin, are certainly known to be successful. Role playing is another effective method, particularly when teaching new communication skills. If the need for advocacy skills has been identified as a learning need, role playing is an ideal method. In participative learning the learner is responsible for acquiring and actualizing the affective, cognitive, and behavioral changes that learning entails, and the teacher provides the means for this process.

In this discussion of participative learning, the lecture method is not ignored, because in some situations it is ideal. Many older adults may be more comfortable with this strategy. The use of supplementary printed materials, such as outlines and notes, should enhance the learning process.

Opportunity for successful learning is provided

In the early contacts with the patient, the practitioner should determine what constitutes positive reinforcement and then use the methods to promote feelings of success. The practitioner should establish short-term achievable goals for each session with the patient. What does the patient specifically want to learn today? New learning should relate to past experiences. If the older person was involved in some physical activity when younger and now must begin a modified exercise program, the practitioner should relate the two experiences. Providing frequent opportunities for feedback also makes older adults feel good about themselves, a factor that motivates learning. Feedback also helps to indicate whether the person is receiving the message as intended.

Problem-centered learning has relevance for older adults

The older person confronted with the need to learn about medications to control chronic illness must recognize the existence of the illness before learning will occur. When the person reaches this stage of acceptance of the illness, teaching is appropriate and desirable. The person then is concerned, seeks and expects immediate answers to present problems, and learning becomes very meaningful.

Application of new knowledge during or immediately after the learning experience enhances the learning process

The adult comes to the setting wanting to learn a new skill that will be useful immediately. Providing an immediate opportunity to practice administration of insulin or explain the new medicine regimen will enhance learning and provide immediate reinforcement.

Teaching is scheduled at a time that is most effective for the older person

Factors that need to be considered in scheduling a teaching session include the person's energy level, attention span, other activities in which the person is involved, availability of family members, and personal preference. Many older persons have a peak time of the day that is generally an effective time for learning to occur.

Appropriate media are used to enhance the learning process

The selection of media used for teaching older adults is critical, primarily because of the wide variety available today. Since most of this population grew up at a time when audiovisual teaching aids were nonexistent, the professional should ask the older adults how they prefer to learn. If they learned through reading and discussion with a teacher during their school years, they may prefer this method. Other persons may have been exposed to other ways of learning through television and may prefer this approach. Because these other methods for learning allow self-pacing and are geared to individualized learning, they may be ideal for the older person. However, this method may be unfamiliar and require the practitioner to thoroughly orient the person to its use.

When selecting any type of medium, the practitioner should use the following criteria:

Large boldface print is used.

Bright, contrasting colors are used, but not green, blue, or violet.

Glossy surfaces are eliminated.

Message is concisely stated.

Terminology is understandable.

Pace is reasonable or controlled by learner.

Small group sessions may facilitate the learning

Older adults need to be carefully assessed in regard to their readiness for small group sessions. They may feel insecure and threatened by a group, or they may be highly responsive. The small group allows each person to contribute and share resources, and much learning can take place from group members as well as from the leader. There are also opportunities to form a peer network in which relationships can be sustained and supported. Some of the learning that can result in a group session may include new attitudes, new solutions to old problems, decreased tension that comes as a result of the support from the group, or perhaps a chance to develop some risk-taking behavior through active participation.

Concepts are presented in a simple and concise manner

In situations in which there is extraneous material older adults have difficulty identifying what is important. They have trouble sorting it out and frequently do not understand abstract ideas. Therefore the material should be briefly and concretely stated in understandable language.

Written information reinforces the learning process

Considerable work that has been done on compliance behavior of older adults indicates that written instructions supplemented by verbal instructions promote greater compliance in taking medications. This principle is applicable to other aspects of learning. Providing the person with an outline of the material to be presented, or perhaps highlights of the program, ensures more effective learning, particularly if the learner refers to it both during the session and later. It also proves to be a useful tool when shared with other health professionals who may be caring for the person, and it is a helpful reference for family members.

Teaching at a slower pace achieves greater learning

Teaching at a slower pace and allowing sufficient time for the person to respond will help the learning process in older adults. Also, if a person is permitted to pace the instruction, ability to comprehend and respond improves. The speed of instruction is an important variable in the learning process.

EVALUATION OF THE LEARNER AND THE PROGRAM

Evaluation and feedback are necessary in the teaching-learning situation for the learner as well as for the professional. The older adult needs feedback on performance from the instructor, so that correct behaviors are reinforced. As indicated previously, verbal compliments or possibly more tangible rewards are motivators for learning. The teacher also needs to be evaluated so the approach can be modified as needed to help the older adult meet previously established objectives.

Evaluation of each person should occur with regularity, to make alterations as well as to provide immediate feedback. The feedback should correct the behavior or reinforce it as it occurs. The evaluation process should be positive. In some situations older adults can be helped to analyze their own behavior; learning can therefore occur when the teacher is not present. Evaluation that occurs at the end of a program is an indication of overall learning that occurs. However, if an attempt is made to identify whether long-term behavioral changes have occurred, an evaluation after an extended period can be planned.

Methods used to evaluate learning in older adults include the traditional written pretest and posttest, comparing knowledge before and after the teaching session. The instructor should carefully explain the purpose of this method, informing the person that test results will guide the teacher in identifying areas of learning needs. If the testing method is used, the materials must be in large, bold print on contrasting paper; the questions should require simple answers; and there must be adequate lighting to compensate for impaired vision.

Another method that is successful is audiotaping the questions and answers. In testing psychomotor learning, the return demonstration has proven successful. If facilities are available, videotaping a psychomotor skill and evaluating it with or without the patient present, serves as an evaluation tool and a learning experience if the patient is present.

ASSESSING LEARNING NEEDS CONCERNING MEDICATION

Before developing a teaching program, the health professional needs to carefully assess the patient's understanding and use of medications. The nurse should also do a thorough health assessment, which will provide baseline information useful in the program planning process. These data should be shared with other practitioners if the data are relevant to their roles in the care of the patient.

Medication history

An area that requires investigation before teaching is started is the medication history, which can be done by the nurse or pharmacist, according to the circumstance and the setting. The pharmacist will focus on the identification of the drugs, expected actions, frequency of administration, and side effects. The nurse is likely to include similar areas plus previous patterns of use of medications, attitudes toward medication, disabilities that may affect administration, and ethnic and religious influences on the treatment of illness. However, because of the expanded teaching roles of these members of the health team, either the nurse or pharmacist may take the full history. The discussion that follows and the specific guidelines are applicable to both groups of practitioners.

If patients are contacted in the home, hospital outpatient, or pharmacy setting, they should be requested to bring all medications with them to facilitate greater accuracy in taking a history. Medications include prescription drugs, over-the-counter drugs, and home remedies. Before the information is gathered, a careful explanation with examples of these three groups is necessary, because over-the-counter drugs and home remedies are not always viewed as medications. Examples of over-the-counter medications include laxatives, antacids, aspirin, and vitamins; examples of home remedies are baking soda for indigestion and lemon juice for colds. When the person brings the medications, the professional also has the opportunity to identify outdated drugs and the use of multiple care providers, which may increase the risk of drug interactions. In taking the medication history, it is suggested that the nurse or pharmacist begin with the prescription drugs, since the patient understands them as medications, and then proceed to the over-the-counter drugs and finally to the home remedies.

After the completion of the history, a careful analysis of problem areas as well as strengths is essential. In situations in which a medication profile is available, it can be used for validation, and the history can supplement the profile. This analysis of the expanded medication history provides data to begin teaching older persons about the wise use of medications.

The following guidelines will assist the practitioner.

Guidelines for taking the medication history

1. Information that the older adult should know about the medication:
   a. What is the name and dose of this drug?

    b. What do you expect the medication to do for you? When should this occur?
    c. When do you take your medication?
    d. How do you take your medication (e.g., with meals, with juice or milk, at bedtime)?
    e. What precautions should you use when taking this medication (e.g., avoid driving, avoid drinking, weigh yourself daily)?
    f. How do you store the medication (e.g., refrigerated, dark container)?
2. Use of memory aids to ensure accuracy in taking drugs:
    a. How do you remember to take your medication as it has been prescribed?
    b. Do you use any special containers or charts to enable you to remember?
    c. Do you carry a card with you that states the name of the drug, dosage, side effects, and name of physician or other practitioner who prescribed it?
3. Factors to assess potential misuse:
    a. Does the patient have any visual, hearing, or memory deficits?
    b. Do physical disabilities possibly interfere with drug administration (e.g., arthritic weakness)?
    c. What are the attitudes of the patient's family toward taking the drug?
    d. Are there economic restrictions that may prevent purchase or affect dose?
    e. Does the patient understand the questions asked?
    f. Does the patient have someone to assist or supervise with administration of the drug?
    g. Does an established routine allow taking the drug at the correct time?
    h. What effects will taking the medication have on life-style?
    i. Are the risks of altering doses, trading drugs with friends, and not reporting side effects understood?
4. Additional factors to assess concerning specific teaching:
    a. What learning method does the patient prefer?
    b. What level of formal education has the patient achieved?
    c. Does the patient recognize taking medications as a problem?
    d. What does the patient view as important to learn?

DEVELOPING A TEACHING PLAN FOR SPECIFIC MEDICATIONS

In developing a lesson plan, the practitioner who has previously assessed the person's learning needs will identify measurable objectives, develop a content outline, determine a method of evaluation, and prepare resources to use during the session. The outline of a teaching plan incorporating these components follows. The plan can be easily adapted for other medications by making changes that are specific to the drugs.

TEACHING PLAN

Class: Teaching older adults about thiazide diuretics
Method: Lecture-discussion

  I. Objectives. At the conclusion of the lesson, the patient:
    A. States the expected drug action
    B. Lists three side effects of medication

   C. Identifies correct action if major side effects occur
   D. Describes one variable to monitor
   E. States three signs of potassium loss
   F. Selects five foods rich in potassium
   G. States dosage and time of administration
   H. Describes correct action if a dose is omitted
II. Lesson plan
   A. Name of medication
   B. Drug action
   C. Side effects
     1. Define meaning of term
     2. List significant side effects
     3. Indicate those requiring immediate action
     4. Identify action to be taken
   D. Potassium loss
     1. State why it occurs
     2. Identify signs of potassium loss
     3. List measures to supplement
       a. Use of potassium when prescribed
       b. Foods rich in potassium
   E. Monitoring
     1. Define meaning in this context
     2. Describe specific activity
   F. Storage of medication
   G. Taking the medication
     1. Identify dose
     2. Identify times of administration
     3. Indicate correct action for missed dose
     4. State importance of taking medication even though patient feels well
   H. Summary and questions
III. Evaluation
   A. Test based on objectives
   B. Discussion based on objectives
IV. Suggested resources
   A. Charts, chalkboard, or overhead transparencies
     1. List of side effects with asterisks marking those requiring immediate action
     2. Telephone with phone numbers listed for physician, pharmacist, nurse
     3. Person in three positions: lying down, sitting up, and standing
     4. List of symptoms of potassium loss
     5. Pictures of potassium-rich foods
     6. Medication label with necessary information
   B. Objectives and outline of class for each participant

PLANNING A COMMUNITY DRUG EDUCATION PROGRAM

Because of the constraints placed on individualized teaching programs, the practitioner-educator can reach a larger number of elderly persons through carefully planned community education programs. Pharmacists and nurses, working individually or collaboratively, have access to older adult populations living independently in senior or private housing and golden age and similar senior groups.

In planning a drug education program, the practitioner will achieve a greater degree of success if a survey is done regarding problems encountered by older adults.

What kinds of questions do people ask about drugs? What information is collected in drug histories? What problems do public health nurses encounter on home visits? Questions of this nature can form the basis for program development.

Older adults make up 11% of the population in the United States and are found everywhere. Suggestions for population groups include residents of independent-living senior housing, senior citizen organizations and centers, neighborhoods with a high percentage of older adults, and church groups. Meeting informally with representatives of these groups will help to determine group needs, scheduling, site for the sessions, and publicity. Programs scheduled at a consistent time, in the same place, and under the sponsorship of an organization lend credence to the program. Before this meeting the planners will need administrative approval if an institution is involved.

The objectives of the programs, preferably based on the needs of the group, or in some cases drawn from the literature, form the basis for program planning. An overall objective, such as to increase the ability of older persons to use medications wisely, will be more clearly defined when specific objectives are established. Examples of specific objectives are: identifies three points on a prescription label that promote safe use, states three side effects of a specified over-the-counter medication (e.g., aspirin), lists two measures to reduce such side effects. The content of the program is defined by the specific objectives.

When the practitioner is planning resources for use with older persons, several criteria previously identified in this chapter must be met. These criteria are significant when selecting and developing materials to be distributed to individual persons or used with the large group. Drug education has proven more successful when handouts supplement the discussion. Drug firms and health education agencies should also be consulted for prepared material.

A drug education program can be evaluated by the amount of group participation, group attentiveness, and interest generated. However, measurement of these factors is very subjective. Development and use of a pre- and posttest is a more objective measurement of new learning. When these tests are developed, the criteria for development of resources are applicable.

A careful explanation of the purpose of the test and the use of terminology other than tests is advisable. To many persons, tests measure success or failure, and the concern for failure within a group is ever-present. Terms such as "survey of understanding of drugs" are less threatening. Another effective method of collecting these evaluation data is to have the health professional available for individual counseling following the program.

SUMMARY

The teaching-learning strategies explored in this chapter will be useful in teaching older adults about medications and other aspects of health promotion. They can be adapted to individuals and groups when teaching about nutrition, exercise, and body changes associated with aging and when coping with these changes and the diseases encountered by older populations.

Nurses, pharmacists, and other practitioners can combine their expertise to provide educational programs in institutions, such as hospitals and nursing homes, and in community sites such as pharmacies, senior centers, senior housing, churches, neighborhood centers, and patient's homes. Carefully designed programs can have a positive effect on the health of older citizens. All health practitioners share the responsibility of helping this group to learn more about themselves so they can function at an optimum level.

SUGGESTED READINGS

Barger, R.C., and Barger, J.: Pharmacist, nurse cooperate in taking drug histories, Hospitals **50**:93, 1976.

Bille, D.A.: Educational strategies for teaching the elderly patient, Nurs. Health Care **1**:256, 1980.

Bozian, M.W., and Clark, H.M.: Counteracting sensory changes in the aging, Am. J. Nurs. **80**:473, 1980.

Hallburg, J.C.: The teaching of aged adults, J. Gerontol. Nurs. **2**(3):13, 1976.

Kim, K., and Grier, M.: Pacing effects of medication instruction for the elderly, J. Gerontol. Nurs. **7**(8):464, 1981.

Lundin, D.: Medication taking behavior of the elderly, Drug Intell. Clin. Pharm. **12**:518, 1978.

Pierce, P.M.: Intelligence and learning in the aged, J. Gerontol. Nurs. **6**(5):268, 1980.

Price, E.: Health education for seniors, Medical Association of the State of Alabama, Dec. 1979.

Pyle, N.: Health education for the aging, J. Gerontol. Nurs. **5**(3):24, 1979.

Schwartz, D.: Safe self-medication for elderly patients, Am. J. Nurs. **75**:1808, 1975.

Stern, E.J.: Helping the person with low vision, Am. J. Nurs. **80**:1788, 1980.

Thorson, J., and Thorson, J.: Patient education and the older drug taker, J. Drug Issues **9**:85, 1979.

Todd, B.: What does a good drug history include? Geriatr. Nurs. **2**:63, 1981.

8

MANAGEMENT OF SELECTED NEUROEMOTIONAL PROBLEMS

Neuroemotional problems in older persons can be very disabling, having an effect on relationships with families, friends, and health practitioners. Depression, anxiety, and insomnia, which are fairly common in older persons, can be relieved by drug therapy when used as an adjunct to emotional support therapy. Parkinson's disease, an incapacitating health problem, is also included in this chapter. Alzheimer's disease has been excluded because of the lack of effective drug treatment.

DEPRESSION

Depression is the most common emotional illness associated with old age. It increases in frequency and degree as the person feels the losses that are incurred when growing older. It is estimated that more than half the people who have a serious depression in their life will have the first episode after the age of 60. Statistics indicate that in persons living in the community the illness is twice as common in older women, a difference that could be attributed to their longer life expectancy. However, in this same population, the suicide rate is three to four times higher for older men (Libow and Sherman, 1981). Unfortunately, depression is frequently mistaken for part of the normal aging process, the depression deepens, and the person does not seek treatment.

Depression is defined as an emotional reaction, a change in mood state, and a group of physical and emotional symptoms that are accompanied by low self-esteem, a negative self-concept, and feelings of helplessness and hopelessness. The affective disorder has been categorized into several types: exogenous and endogenous, situational and clinical, unipolar and bipolar. A generalized concept of depression will be included in this section.

The causes of depression have been cited as stressful life events, disturbances in physical health, and the general losses associated with aging. Some of the losses of old age include physical energy and stamina, memory, sensory abilities, sources of intimacy and friendship, and decreased status and income associated with employment, home, and general health. Any of these losses, or a combination, may contribute to a depressive reaction.

Attention has been given to the role of chemicals in the brain that help regulate nervous system activity. Butler and Lewis (1982) report two classes of chemicals that are important in depression: catecholamines, which include dopamine and norepinephrine, and serotonin. Because these transmitters are decreased when depression exists, it is postulated that this decline may be a factor in the cause of depression. Pharmacological therapy has been based on the deficits of these neurotransmitters, although evidence is lacking to substantiate this theory.

Additional factors known to cause depression in older persons include chronic illnesses, especially those that are debilitating such as Parkinson's disease and stroke. The use of medications such as antihypertensives, antiparkinsonian drugs, antipsychotic drugs, and glucocorticoids may also be a factor causing depression in the older adult.

Signs and symptoms

The major signs and symptoms of depression are well known and felt in varying degrees by many individuals. The extremes are transient "blues" to frank psychoses to suicide. Physiological signs common to depression include anorexia, weight loss, constipation, tachycardia, fatigue, insomnia, decreased libido, and agitation or psychomotor retardation. Psychological symptoms include feeling sad or "blue"; crying; feelings of emptiness, hopelessness, and helplessness; indecisiveness; inability to concentrate; expressions of guilt and anger; personal devaluation; and thoughts of suicide.

Depression has been diagnosed by using the dexamethasone suppression test, which is conducted by giving 1 mg dexamethasone at 11 PM and measuring serum cortisol at 4 PM and 11 PM the next day. Serum cortisol is depressed following dexamethasone administration in normal individuals but remains at normal levels in patients with depression. This test is approximately 50% effective in diagnosing "endogenous" depression.

The rate of suicide in the older population is an indication of the urgent need for intervention by qualified health practitioners. The general suicide rate in the United States is 10/100,000 people, which increases to 150/100,000 for elderly divorced, white males in their 70s (Busse and Pfeiffer, 1977). Suicidal attempts are carefully planned and generally successful. The highest rate of suicide occurs in white males who are over 80 years of age. The danger of suicide makes treatment imperative.

Management

A variety of treatment modalities are effective in helping the depressed person. A thorough evaluation is recommended to determine possible causes, such as medications and physical problems. We recognize the importance of psychotherapy and other therapies; however, this section will deal only with the antidepressant medications used to treat depression.

Tricyclic antidepressants

Tricyclic antidepressants are the drugs most widely used in the treatment of depression. Despite their pharmacological and chemical similarity, the drugs differ in sedative and anticholinergic effects, norepinephrine and serotonin activity, potency, dosage, and individual effects (Fischer and Kroboth, 1980). Commonly used tricyclic antidepressants are amitriptyline, desipramine, doxepin, imipramine, amoxapine, maprotiline, and trimipramine. The medications will be discussed as a class with attention to individual variations when appropriate.

Drug action. The mechanism of the antidepressant action of tricyclic antidepressants is not certain, because the biological nature of depression is not clear. It is postulated that in depression a functional deficiency of biogenic amines (dopamine, tryptamine, norepinephrine, and serotonin) exists at the postsynaptic adrenergic receptors in the brain. They are stored in storage vesicles in the presynaptic neuron, and on stimulation, the vesicles secrete an amount of amine into the synapse. These amine substances diffuse across the synapse, producing conduction along the postsynaptic neuron by stimulating its receptors. The stimulation is terminated by reuptake of the amines into the presynaptic neuron. The tricyclic antidepressants inhibit this reuptake, thereby increasing the concentration of this neurotransmitter. The drugs differ in their ability to block the specific neurotransmitters. The general availability of methods to determine levels of serotonin and norepinephrine will facilitate the selection of the tricyclic antidepressant most effective for a specific deficiency.

All the tricyclic antidepressants are highly lipid soluble and are readily absorbed from the gastrointestinal tract. Interactions are common because the drugs are highly protein bound. They are metabolized by liver enzymes, and approximately two thirds are excreted in the urine and one third in the feces. Plasma levels of imipramine, amitriptyline, and desipramine increase with age for patients who are on a fixed dosage, and this increase indicates the need for a lower dosage. Lower dosage may also decrease cardiotoxic and CNS side effects in the older patient.

Since all tricyclic antidepressants have therapeutic half-lives longer than 24 hours, once-a-day bedtime dosing is possible when the dose has been stabilized and if it is tolerated by the patient. Once-a-day dosing is advantageous because the patient is asleep and unaware of the annoying side effects, less mental and physical impairment occurs during the day, compliance is better, and the use of a hypnotic is usually unnecessary, since maximum use of the sedative properties of these drugs is made. Patients who cannot tolerate a single bedtime dose can usually be given one third to one half the dose after the evening meal and the rest at bedtime.

The increased sensitivity of older adults to anticholinergic effects of medications should be a factor in product selection. Anticholinergic effects are greatest with amitriptyline, moderate with imipramine, nortriptyline, and doxepin, and least with desipramine (Salzman, 1979). Sedative effects are greatest with doxepin, moderate with amitriptyline and imipramine, and least with desipramine. Doxepin produces little hypotension and cardiotoxicity and modest anticholinergic effects.

Drug	Dosage*
Amitriptyline	75 to 300 mg/day.
Desipramine	75 to 300 mg/day.
Doxepin	75 to 300 mg/day.
Imipramine	75 to 300 mg/day.
Trimipramine	75 to 200 mg/day.
Amoxapine	150 to 300 mg/day.
Maprotiline (tetracyclic)	75 to 225 mg/day.

Proper use and precautions
1. Medication should be taken with food to decrease the possibility of gastric upset.
2. Taking medications at bedtime enhances sedative effects. If nightmares or postural hypotension occurs, a half dose should be taken at bedtime and the remainder during the day.
3. Small doses (one third to one half of the usual adult dose) are recommended in initial therapy with small increments until the optimum dose is achieved. Liquid dosage forms may be used to provide for smaller doses.
4. Optimum effects of the medication may not occur for 4 to 6 weeks.
5. Medication should not be discontinued without discussing the change with the physician.
6. Before the patient undergoes any type of surgery, the physician or dentist should be notified about this medication.
7. Drugs must be kept out of reach of children, because overdose is particularly dangerous with them.
8. Because medication may affect alertness, the patient should exercise caution about driving and using household or job-related mechanical equipment.

*One-third to one-half dose is recommended for initial therapy in geriatric patients.

9. Drinking alcohol must be avoided while taking these drugs.
10. If the medication is taken in oral liquid form, it should not be mixed with grape juice or carbonated beverages, since this may decrease effectiveness.
11. Because dizziness, light-headedness, and fainting may occur, the patient should be advised to rise slowly from lying to sitting to standing position.
12. Drug interactions that may occur include alcohol and other CNS depressants (CNS depression), anticonvulsants (CNS depression and decreased effect of anticonvulsants), guanethidine (blocking of antihypertensive effects), MAO inhibitors (possible hyperpyretic crisis, convulsions, and death), sympathomimetics (possible severe hypertension and hyperpyrexia).
13. Side effects that may occur include blurred vision, constipation, urinary retention, irregular heartbeat, slow pulse, dizziness, fainting, delirium, tremors, dry mouth, nausea, and increased appetite for sweets.
14. Monitoring includes regular physician visits, blood cell counts, hepatic function determinations, cardiac function monitoring, and blood pressure determinations.

Trazodone

Drug action. Trazodone is chemically unrelated to tricyclic, tetracyclic, or other known antidepressant drugs. The mechanism of action is not well understood, but the drug is thought to selectively inhibit serotonin uptake by brain receptors at the synapse. Response to therapy occurs in 2 weeks in most patients. This drug is reported to have fewer anticholinergic and cardiovascular side effects.

Drug	Dosage
Trazodone	100 to 400 mg/day.

Proper use and precautions
1. Medication should be taken with or shortly after a meal to decrease the risk of dizziness and light-headedness.
2. Sedative effects may require most of the dose to be given at bedtime.
3. Medication should not be discontinued without discussing the change with the physician.
4. Before the patient undergoes any type of surgery, the physician or dentist should be notified about this medication.
5. Because medication may affect alertness, the patient should exercise caution about driving and using household or job-related mechanical equipment.

6. Drug interactions that may occur include alcohol and other CNS depressants (CNS depression) and antihypertensives (hypotension).
7. Side effects that may occur include drowsiness, dizziness, fatigue, blurred vision, constipation, and dry mouth.
8. Monitoring includes regular physician visits, white blood cell and differential counts, and cardiac function tests.

ANXIETY

The stresses of society are reflected in the behavior of older persons who frequently experience various levels of anxiety. This behavior may have been a lifelong pattern, or it may occur for the first time in the later years. The causes of anxiety are many and may include the losses associated with aging, increasing dependency, and the constant need for adaptations in coping behavior.

Signs and symptoms

The symptoms of anxiety in younger persons may appear in older persons also but more often are not manifested in the pure form. Anxiety, which occurs in response to some vague internal problem the person may not be aware of, is more likely to be associated with depression or hypochondriasis. However, the practitioner must be alert for nervous feelings, muscle and motor phenomena, and autonomic responses. The older person does not respond to anxiety as do younger persons, who demonstrate fright-flight behavior. Instead, they may demonstrate fright-freeze behavior, which can have a more devastating impact on the body without the release of tension felt by younger persons.

Management

The benzodiazepines are considered the preferred drugs for the treatment of anxiety in older adults because there is less interference with the metabolism of other drugs, length of action of the drug indicates that a single daily dose is satisfactory, and the drug is less apt to cause physical dependency (Lamy, 1980).

Benzodiazepines

Drug action. The sites and mechanisms of action of the benzodiazepines are uncertain, but they appear to enhance presynaptic inhibition through a GABA-ergic (gamma aminobutyric acid) mechanism. Therefore selected actions of the drug are decreased by agents that either decrease the synthesis or antagonize GABA and increased by agents that increase local GABA concentrations. The drugs are used as sedative-hypnotics as well as antianxiety agents. As a group, they are less sedating and cause less mental clouding than do the barbiturates or other hypnotics. Members of the group vary in duration of action, with lorazepam and oxazepam having relatively short durations of action, diazepam a moderate duration, and prazepam a long duration of action. Drugs with a shorter duration of action are less sedating.

Drug	Dosage
Alprazolam	0.75 to 1.5 mg/day.
Chlorazepate monopotassium	13 to 52 mg/day.
Chlorazepate dipotassium	15 to 60 mg/day.
Chlordiazepoxide	15 to 100 mg/day.
Diazepam	5 to 60 mg/day.
Lorazepam	1 to 6 mg/day.
Oxazepam	30 to 120 mg/day.
Prazepam	20 to 60 mg/day.

Proper use and precautions
1. Medication should be taken only as directed and not discontinued without consultation with the physician.
2. Because the medication may cause dizziness, drowsiness, and decreased alertness, the patient should understand its effects before operating a car, machinery, or dangerous household equipment.
3. The medication should be used with caution for patients with the following medical problems: drug abuse, depression, epilepsy, hepatic function or renal impairment, narrow-angle glaucoma, and pulmonary disease.
4. Dependency may occur.
5. Drug interactions may occur with the following drugs: alcohol, anesthetics, CNS depressants, MAO inhibitors, or tricyclic antidepressants (concurrent use may increase effects of either medication), and cimetidine (sedative effects may increase).
6. Side effects may include light-headedness; drowsiness; fatigue; headache; ataxia; depression; blurred vision; skin rash; unusual excitement, nervousness, or irritability (paradoxical reaction); or bradycardia or breathing problems (CNS depression).
7. Monitoring includes regular physician visits when the patient is taking the medication for an extended period, blood cell counts, hepatic function determination, and assessment of drug effectiveness.

PSYCHOSES

The following brief discussion of the major tranquilizers is included because psychotic people grow old, psychosis can occur in older persons, and psychotic persons may be encountered living in both the community and in nursing homes. An additional reason for inclusion of this group of medications relates to tardive dyskinesia, a syndrome associated with long-term use of this group of drugs. A discussion of psychiatric illness will not be included in this section, and the reader is directed to psychiatric literature.

Management

The use of antipsychotic drugs for older persons must be carefully evaluated against the hazard of causing tardive dyskinesia. Butler and Lewis (1982) report that chronic schizophrenia is the major condition for which drugs are clinically justified on a long-term basis. They recommend that the drugs be administered with caution in older people, beginning with low doses, and very gradually increased only when a higher dose is indicated. The patient must be observed by skilled practitioners who are aware of the potential dangers of the medication. The potential dangers, complications, and side effects of the medications should be discussed with the patient and family.

Antipsychotic drugs that may be useful for elderly persons and will be discussed in this section include the phenothiazines and butyrophenones.

Antipsychotic drugs
Phenothiazines and butyrophenones

Drug action. The exact mechanism of drug action is not fully understood, but evidence indicates that the drug affects the transmission of nerve impulses in CNS pathways in which the neurotransmitter is the catecholamine dopamine. The drug acts by blockading the postsynaptic neurons or inhibiting the neurotransmitter release from postsynaptic nerve impulses and thereby interfering with the transmission of impulses in the limbic and extrapyramidal systems. The resultant action when the drug is administered to psychotic patients is a tranquilizing or sedative effect and an antipsychotic effect or a normalizing of mood, thought, and behavior. The drugs are used in schizophrenia and other psychiatric disorders and in the control of anxiety, restlessness, and agitation.

Drug	Dosage
Phenothiazines	
Chlorpromazine	10 to 1000 mg/day.
Trifluoperazine	2 to 20 mg/day.

Drug	Dosage
Thioridazine	20 to 200 mg/day.
Numerous others	
Butyrophenone	
Haloperidol	1 to 15 mg/day.

Proper use and precautions
1. Small doses are recommended, particularly with the frail elderly, who may have a marked sensitivity to the drug.
2. The effects of the medication may not be achieved for several weeks.
3. The medication is to be taken exactly as prescribed and should not be discontinued without consultation with the physician, because withdrawal symptoms may occur.
4. Before the patient undergoes any type of surgery, the physician or dentist should be notified about this medication.
5. The medication should be taken with food or a full glass of water or milk to reduce gastric irritation.
6. If the medication is measured with a dropper, it should be diluted with half a glass of tomato or fruit juice, milk, or carbonated beverage.
7. The medication should not be taken within an hour of taking antacids or antidiarrheal medication.
8. If a liquid form of the medication is being administered, care should be taken to avoid getting it on the skin, because it may cause a rash.
9. Because the medication may cause drowsiness, the patient should exercise caution about driving and using household or job-related mechanical equipment.
10. If dizziness, drowsiness, or fainting occurs when changing positions, the patient should be advised to rise very slowly to a standing position.
11. Because the medication decreases perspiration and the ability of the body to cool itself, care must be exercised to avoid overheating in exercise, hot weather, and hot baths.
12. Sun sensitivity may occur, so precautions should be taken, particularly when beginning the medication.
13. Alcohol and other CNS depressant drugs should not be taken concurrently.
14. Medication may cause urine to turn reddish brown.
15. Drug interactions may occur with alcohol or other CNS depressants (potentiate or prolong effects), antacids or antidiarrheals (may affect absorption), anticonvulsants (may lower seizure threshold), anticholinergics (affect action of both drugs), epinephrine (may cause

severe hypotension), guanethidine (may block antihypertensive effects), levodopa (may block antiparkinsonian effects), MAO inhibitors or tricyclic antidepressants (may exaggerate sedative and anticholinergic effects).

16. Side effects that are possible with any phenothiazine include muscle spasms of neck and back; restlessness; shuffling gait; ticlike movements of head, face, mouth, and neck; trembling of hands and fingers; flycatcher tongue movement; skin rash; eye changes; sore throat; yellowing of eyes and skin; hypotension; decreased sweating; photosensitivity; blurred vision; constipation; dry mouth; nasal congestion; difficult urination; and decreased sexual ability. Often an anticholinergic drug is prescribed to decrease extrapyramidal side effects.

COMPARISON OF SIDE EFFECTS OF PHENOTHIAZINES

Name	Sedation	Hypotension	Extrapyramidal effects
Chlorpromazine	Marked	Occasional	Occasional
Thioridazine	Moderate	Moderate	Infrequent
Trifluoperazine	Minimum	Minimum	Frequent

17. Specific comments about haloperidol: actions, indications, and adverse effects are similar to the phenothiazines. However, sedation and hypotension may be less common than with chlorpromazine, and extrapyramidal symptoms are similar to trifluoperazine.
18. Monitoring includes regular physician visits, monitoring of drug effectiveness, careful observation for tardive dyskinesia, blood cell counts, liver function tests, and ophthalmic examination (with high-dose or prolonged therapy).

Tardive dyskinesia. Tardive dyskinesia, a syndrome associated mainly with the antipsychotics, primarily the phenothiazines and butyrophenones, has become increasingly prevalent in older persons. Elderly people who have been treated with these medications for confusion, agitation, depression, and other psychiatric-type illnesses are particularly vulnerable to tardive dyskinesia. It occurs more commonly in females and in persons with a history of brain damage. The syndrome may or may not diminish when the medication is withdrawn, but irreversibility occurs almost exclusively in the older adult (Portnoi and Johnson, 1982).

Manifestations of tardive dyskinesia are generally clear, and the health practitioner can readily identify the problem. Abnormal facial movements may be the first symptoms to be observed. Puffing of the cheeks, smacking and pursing of the lips, lateral jaw movements, "flycatcher" movement of the tongue, and problems of chewing and swallowing are evident. Rhythmic and involuntary movements of trunk and limbs may include jerking of the extremities, rubbing body parts, and constant hand and foot movement. The movements vary in intensity and body parts affected. The symptoms of tardive dyskinesia should not be confused with the voluntary actions such as motor restlessness that are associated with the antipsychotics.

Treatment of tardive dyskinesia has been varied, with no therapy particularly effective. Careful vigilance for the appearance of the symptoms, with subsequent withdrawal of the medication, is recommended. Periodic review of drug therapy by the health team also functions as a measure of prevention.

INSOMNIA

In recent years the subject of sleep has received considerable attention, but limited attention has been focused on the effect of aging on the sleep process. However, it is known that older adults have sleep disturbances in various forms. The total duration of sleep may remain the same or less, but the quality of sleep undergoes the most change. Both the number and length of wakeful periods increase, and this change can be the most distressing.

Signs and symptoms

The change in sleep patterns and the incidence of insomnia as reported by older persons may have a variety of causes. Recent retirement or a change in life-style may be a factor; the person rearranges the sleep cycle by sleeping later in the morning, taking naps during the day, and then going to bed at the usual time, which may be too early. Symptoms associated with physical health problems that may be disturbing sleep patterns include joint pain, cough, dyspnea, and nocturia. Treatment of the illness causing the symptom can improve sleep patterns. The emotional concerns of this period of life, with the associated worry behavior, also contribute to alterations in sleep patterns.

Management

If the health professional is in a position to take a sleep history, inquiring about the specific sleeping patterns, recent life-style changes, and factors that promote or hinder sleep can be very beneficial in offering suggestions to enhance the sleep process and also in the selection of a sedative-hypnotic.

The use of sedative-hypnotics is questionable because many of these drugs disrupt normal sleeping patterns; have side effects such as oversedation, incontinence, hypotension, and paradoxical stimulation; and result in physical dependency. Flurazepam and chloral hydrate have been selected for discussion in this section because they cause the least disturbance in the older person's sleep cycle. Barbiturates have been excluded because of their adverse effects on elderly patients.

Sedative-hypnotics
Flurazepam

Drug action. See antianxiety agents—Benzodiazepines. Flurazepam induces sleep rapidly and has been found effective for most sleep disorders, allowing the patient a full night of sleep.

Drug	Dosage
Flurazepam	15 to 30 mg; increased dosage in older adults is not recommended because of the increased risk of oversedation.

Proper use and precautions
1. See comments under benzodiazepines.
2. In addition to the previously identified side effects, daytime drowsiness, dizziness, and motor incoordination may occur.

Chloral hydrate

Drug action. Chloral hydrate is a CNS depressant. It is used for elderly patients because it reportedly produces less paradoxical excitement than do barbiturates.

Drug	Dosage
Chloral hydrate	250 to 500 mg.

Proper use and precautions
1. The capsule must be swallowed whole, and it is suggested that a full glass of water, fruit juice, or ginger ale will decrease gastric upset.
2. If the oral liquid form is prescribed, it should be mixed with half a glass of any of the previously mentioned liquids, which will improve flavor and decrease gastric upset.
3. Medication should be taken only as directed and not discontinued without consulting the physician. Rapid withdrawal can result in withdrawal symptoms. Physical dependence can occur.
4. Before the patient undergoes any type of surgery, the physician or dentist should be notified about this medication.
5. The medication should be used with caution for patients with severe cardiac disease, severe renal or hepatic function impairment, and gastritis.
6. Because the medication may cause dizziness, drowsiness, and decreased alertness, the patient should become familiar with its action

before driving a car or operating other dangerous mechanical equipment.

7. The medication may cause false-positive glucose determinations with Benedict's solution and possibly with cupric sulfate tablets but not with glucose enzymatic tests.
8. Drug interactions may occur with alcohol, anesthetics, CNS depressants, MAO inhibitors, or tricyclic antidepressants (may increase effects of either medication) or oral anticoagulants (may increase hypoprothrombinemic effects).
9. Side effects that may occur include shortness of breath and irregular heartbeat (symptoms of overdose), skin rash, hallucinations, unusual excitement, mental confusion, nausea, vomiting, stomach pain, clumsiness, light-headedness, drowsiness, and hangover feeling.
10. Monitoring consists of regular physician visits.

PARKINSON'S DISEASE

Parkinson's disease, a disabling condition, is the most common neurological disorder among older adults. First symptoms generally occur in the sixth decade, with the disease more common in men. It is expected that as the life span lengthens, the incidence of the illness will increase.

Signs and symptoms

The characteristic symptoms of Parkinson's disease occur as a result of changes in the basal ganglia of the cerebrum, which function as neural processing stations for messages. Dopamine, the neurotransmitter substance produced by the substantia nigra, is known to be deficient. As the substantia nigra atrophies, the amount of dopamine diminishes, and the result is a condition characterized by slowness of movement, tremor at rest, and muscular rigidity. The symptoms of Parkinson's disease also occur as a result of therapy with phenothiazine derivatives.

The course of the disease is variable. Symptoms may progress at a very slow rate but are progressive until eventually the person is disabled and unable to provide self-care. The symptoms generally begin unilaterally and progress to bilateral movement. The characteristic pill-rolling tremor is worse at rest and decreased during movement. A second symptom is muscular rigidity that produces a cogwheel effect, which is a jerking, uncoordinated movement. There is generalized muscular stiffness, resulting in weakness and a slowing down process. The gait of persons with Parkinson's disease is characterized by the head being held forward, short, shuffling steps, and lack of general coordinated movement. The disease is further complicated by increased salivation, dysphagia, constipation, and incontinence. Depression and withdrawal behavior are common. Ultimately, severe invalidism occurs, with associated susceptibility to infections and further complications.

Management

Presently, treatment is supportive and symptomatic. Supportive counseling may be advisable for the patient and the caregivers. Maintaining adequate nutrition presents problems, since chewing and swallowing become increasingly more difficult (Fischbach, 1978). Physical activity should be maintained, and the services of a physical therapist may be needed to assist in a program of exercises. Drug therapy, which is directed at reducing muscular rigidity, tremors, and akinesia, has many undesirable side effects. Drugs included in this section are benztropine, trihexyphenidyl, amantadine, bromocriptine, levodopa, and a carbidopa/levodopa combination.

Anticholinergic agents
Benztropine

Drug action. A long-acting medication, benztropine has a central anticholinergic effect that releases skeletal muscular rigidity, cramps, and spasms. The antispasmodic action brings pain relief to patients with Parkinson's disease, and because of an additional sedative effect, it also relieves insomnia. The drug is also used in treating parkinsonism produced by drugs that induce extrapyramidal motor system reactions.

Drug	Dosage
Benztropine mesylate tablets Benztropine mesylate injection	1 to 2 mg one to two times daily, with maximum doses of 6 mg. Small increments are advisable for elderly patients.

Proper use and precautions
1. Medication should be increased in small increments for elderly patients.
2. Medication should be taken at bedtime with food to decrease gastric irritation.
3. Antacids and antidiarrheal medications should be avoided within 1 hour of taking benztropine.
4. Hard sugarless candies, sugarless gum, and ice chips may be taken to relieve the problems associated with dry mouth caused by the medication. Artificial saliva is also beneficial.

5. Alcohol and other CNS depressants must be avoided.
6. Because the medication causes heat intolerance, the patient is advised not to become overheated during hot weather or when exercising or bathing.
7. Because medication may affect alertness, the patient should exercise caution about driving a car or operating household or mechanical equipment.
8. If the eyes become more light sensitive than usual while the medication is being taken, sunglasses are advised.
9. Older or debilitated patients may respond to usual doses with excitement, agitation, drowsiness, or confusion and may require a decreased dose.
10. Drug interactions may occur with amantadine, antihistamines, other anticholinergics, haloperidol, MAO inhibitors, phenothiazines, procainamide, quinidine, tricyclic antidepressants (may intensify atropine-like effects), or antacids or antidiarrheals (may reduce therapeutic effects of benztropine).
11. Side effects that may occur include constipation, difficult urination, eye pain, skin rash, bloated feeling, dizziness, dry mouth, headache, rapid pulse, and reduced sweating. Additional but less frequently occurring side effects are blurred vision, decreased sexual ability, drowsiness, visual light sensitivity, fatigue, confusion, nervousness, and reduced sense of taste.
12. Monitoring includes regular physician visits and determination of intraocular pressure.

Trihexyphenidyl

Drug action. Trihexyphenidyl provides symptomatic relief by reducing skeletal muscle rigidity, lessening tremors, and counteracting akinesia. The drug produces a mild euphoric effect helpful in overcoming depression associated with the disease. The drug is also useful in reducing the extrapyramidal motor system reactions caused by certain drugs.

Drug	Dosage
Trihexyphenidyl extended-release capsules	5 mg daily after breakfast with an additional 5 mg taken 12 hours later as needed.
Trihexyphenidyl elixir or tablets	1 to 2 mg on the first day with increases of 2 mg at 3 to 5 day intervals until dose reaches 10 to 15 mg given in three to four divided doses.

Proper use and precautions. See Benztropine.

Other antiparkinsonian agents
Amantadine

Drug action. The mechanism of amantadine is not clearly understood but may be related to the release of dopamine and other catecholamines from neuronal storage sites or to delayed reuptake of these neurotransmitters into synaptic vesicles; it reduces severity of signs and symptoms in some patients.

Drug	Dosage
Amantadine capsules	100 to 200 mg/day.
Amantadine syrup	

Proper use and precautions
1. See Anticholinergic agents (Benztropine and Trihexyphenidyl) regarding proper use and precautions.
2. Side effects that may occur are similar to the anticholinergics. Additional side effects include depression, orthostatic hypotension, psychosis, peripheral edema, congestive heart failure, anorexia, and nausea.

Levodopa and carbidopa/levodopa

Drug action. The symptoms of Parkinson's disease are caused by insufficient dopamine. However, dopamine does not cross the blood-brain barrier and therefore cannot be used as a replacement drug. Levodopa, which is the metabolic precursor of dopamine, does cross the blood-brain barrier, where it is converted to dopamine by the enzyme dopa decarboxylase. Less than 1% of the absorbed levodopa penetrates the CNS site of action, and the remainder is decarboxylated peripherally to dopamine, which does not cross the blood-brain barrier and is excreted.

Levodopa lessens bradykinesia, rigidity, and tremor. Because the peripheral effects of levodopa cause reactions such as nausea and cardiac arrhythmias, a dopa decarboxylase inhibitor, carbidopa, has been combined with levodopa to block these peripheral effects. By preventing the peripheral metabolism of levodopa, carbidopa increases the amount of levodopa available for decarboxylation to dopamine in the brain. This action produces a therapeutic response with lowered dosage and reduces peripheral side effects, especially nausea.

Drug	Dosage
Levodopa capsules	Initially, 250 mg two to four times daily with daily
Levodopa tablets	dosage increased by 100 to 750 mg at 3 to 7 day intervals as tolerated. Usual prescribing limit is 8 gm/day.

Drug	Dosage
Carbidopa/levodopa tablets	Initially, 10 mg carbidopa and 100 mg levodopa with daily dosage increased by one tablet daily up to six tablets/day. For patients being converted from levodopa, careful titration of dosage is essential. Most patients can be maintained on three to six tablets of 25 mg carbidopa/250 mg levodopa daily; usual prescribing limits are 200 mg carbidopa and 2 gm levodopa/day.

Proper use and precautions

1. Medication is to be taken with solid food to decrease gastric irritation.
2. Full effects of medication may not be achieved for several weeks.
3. Pyridoxine (vitamin B_6) decreases the effects of levodopa. Therefore vitamin products containing it should be avoided unless prescribed. Common foods rich in this vitamin include avocados, bacon, beans, beef liver, dry skim milk, oatmeal, peas, pork, sweet potatoes, and tuna. Restriction of pyridoxine is not necessary with carbidopa.
4. High-protein meals can block the effects of levodopa because of its protein-binding capabilities. Limiting the amount of milk, meat, fish, poultry, cheese, and eggs in the diet is recommended. However, a consistent amount of protein is important for maximum drug effect.
5. Occasionally, dark discoloration of urine may occur, which is insignificant.
6. Patients should be encouraged to rise slowly from lying or sitting positions to counteract the effects of postural hypotension that may be drug induced.
7. Because mental acuity may be altered, patients should be advised to use caution about driving and using household or job-related mechanical equipment.
8. The drug may affect home-testing results of urine for glucose and acetone.
9. As patients begin to feel better, they should be instructed to gradually increase their physical activity as their bodies adapt to changes.
10. Drug interactions may occur with pyridoxine (antagonizes levodopa), antihypertensive agents (increase hypotensive effects), methyldopa (decreases antiparkinsonian effect and increases hypotensive effect), MAO inhibitors (may cause hypertensive crisis), sympathomimetics (may cause cardiac arrhythmias), haloperidol, papaverine, phenothiazines, phenytoin, or reserpine (decreases effects of levodopa).
11. Drug should be used with caution for patients with various conditions that affect older adults, including emphysema, predisposition to nar-

    row-angle glaucoma, impaired renal or hepatic function, and depression.

12. Side effects that may occur are anorexia, nausea and vomiting, dry mouth, burning sensation of tongue, constipation, diarrhea, urinary retention, mood changes (especially depression), unusual and uncontrolled movements of body parts, headache, dizziness, orthostatic hypotension, and cardiac irregularities. Persons receiving this medication for 1 or more years may have sudden, unexpected akinesia, tremor, and rigidity alternated with a phase of dyskinetic movement (on-off response), which may require frequent dosage changes. Nausea and vomiting are reported less frequently with carbidopa.

13. Monitoring includes regular visits to physician, blood cell counts, hepatic function determinations, renal function determinations, cardiovascular monitoring, ophthalmoscopic examinations, and observation for changes in symptoms.

Bromocriptine mesylate

Drug action. Bromocriptine mesylate produces its therapeutic effect by directly stimulating the dopamine receptors in the corpus striatum. Used in conjunction with reduced dosage of carbidopa/levodopa, it extends the period of control with these medications for patients with "end of dose" failure; it is also used for patients unable to tolerate or unresponsive to levodopa therapy.

Drug	Dosage
Bromocriptine mesylate	Initial dosage is 1.25 mg two times daily. Increase by 2.5 mg daily every 2 to 4 weeks only as necessary.

Proper use and precautions

1. See Carbidopa/levodopa.
2. Side effects are similar to carbidopa/levodopa, with the addition of signs and symptoms of ergotism such as tingling of fingers, cold feet, numbness, muscle cramps, and exacerbation of Raynaud's syndrome.

REFERENCES

Busse, E., and Pfeiffer, E.: Behavior and adaptation in late life, Boston, 1977, Little, Brown & Co.

Butler, R.N., and Lewis, M.I.: Aging and mental health: positive psychosocial approaches, ed. 3, St. Louis, 1982, The C.V. Mosby Co.

Fischbach, F.: Easing adjustment of Parkinson's disease, Am. J. Nurs. **78**:66, 1978.

Fischer, J., and Kroboth, P.: Update: tricyclic antidepressant therapy, U.S. Pharmacist **5**:33, April 1980.

Lamy, P.: Prescribing for the elderly, Littleton, Mass., 1980, PSG Publishing Co., Inc.

Libow, L.S., and Sherman, F.T.: The core of geriatric medicine: a guide for students and practitioners, St. Louis, 1981, The C.V. Mosby Co.

Portnoi, V., and Johnson, J.: Tardive dyskinesia, Geriatr. Nurs. **3**(1):3, 1982.
Salzman, C.: Update on geriatric pharmacology, Geriatrics **34:**87, Aug. 1979.

SUGGESTED READINGS

Baptista, R.: The tricyclic antidepressants: a current perspective, Hospital Formulary **16:**724, July 1981.
Burnside, I., editor: Psychosocial nursing care of the aged, ed. 2, New York, 1980, McGraw-Hill Book Co.
Coleman, J., and Dorevitch, A.: Rational use of psychoactive drugs in the geriatric patient, Drug Intell. Clin. Pharm. **15:**940, 1981.
Ebersole, P., and Hess, P.: Toward healthy aging: human needs and nursing response, St. Louis, 1981, The C.V. Mosby Co.
Fitzgerald, C.: Physiological changes affecting drug handling in the aged, J. Gerontol. Nurs. **6:**207, 1980.
Todd, B.: Could your patient's confusion be caused by drugs? Geriatr. Nurs. **2:**291, 1981.
U.S. Department of Health, Education, and Welfare: 1979 FDA Drug Bulletin **9**(2):2, 1979.
U.S. Department of Health, Education, and Welfare: 1979 FDA Drug Bulletin **9**(3):16, 1979.

9

MANAGEMENT OF SELECTED MUSCULOSKELETAL PROBLEMS

Changes affecting the musculoskeletal system have a serious impact on the life-style of the older person. The alterations, caused by normal changes compounded by pathological changes, can be delayed with appropriate management. Recognition of the changes by the older person, consultation with practitioners regarding self-management and the need for medical therapy, and guiding the person in the therapeutic regimen will aid in the prevention of complications.

The problems selected for discussion in this chapter are osteoarthritis, rheumatoid arthritis, gout, and osteoporosis. The major focus of management is drug therapy.

OSTEOARTHRITIS

Osteoarthritis, the most common type of arthritis, affects only 10% of the population under 30, but nearly all persons over 75 have evidence of it. Older persons are particularly vulnerable to the illness because of the aging process, trauma, obesity, and prior inflammatory disease. Women under 60 report the symptoms twice as frequently as men do, but in the older age groups the distribution is equal.

The hallmark of osteoarthritis is cartilage destruction and reparation. The alterations in osteoarthritic cartilage vary from site to site, are localized, and roughly approximate the severity of the disease. Although the cause of osteoarthritis is uncertain, some authorities believe that it occurs as a result of mechanical injury to portions of the articular cartilage of the joint surface.

Signs and symptoms

A slowly progressive, symmetrical disease, osteoarthritis is characterized by pain, stiffness, deformity, and limitation of motion. The pain, frequently described as aching, is the main symptom that occurs on weight bearing and motion. The pain becomes worse with activity and improves with rest; this improvement differentiates it from rheumatoid arthritis. The stiffness, which occurs in the morning or after sitting, disappears more rapidly than in rheumatoid arthritis. The disease process affects the major weight-bearing joints —hips, knees, and cervical, thoracic, and lumbar joints. However, the most commonly affected joints are the hips, knees, first carpometacarpal joints, and distal interphalangeal joints. Crepitation, or a grating sound, can often be heard as the joint is put through range of motion. Heberden's nodes are bony enlargements that occur at the distal interphalangeal joints of the hands. The nodes are potentially deforming, are most common in women, and tend to run in families.

Management

The treatment of osteoarthritis is primarily symptomatic. Aspirin and mild analgesics are used for pain relief. Medication taken at regular intervals will prevent severe pain and permit the person to participate in physical activities. A regular program of rest and activity, possibly supplemented by physical therapy (heat, ultrasound, and massage), will promote comfort. Weight reduction and correction of factors that cause strain are advised.

RHEUMATOID ARTHRITIS

Rheumatoid arthritis is a chronic, systemic disease characterized by bilateral symmetrical joint inflammation. In the United States, approximately 2% to 3% of the population has the disease, which is more common in women than men. However, after the age of 80, the male-female distribution is equal. Onset of the disease generally occurs between 20 and 60 years and peaks between 25 and 45, but the initial attack can occur in older people. The course of illness in old persons is often relentless despite treatment, possibly because of an ineffective immune system. The incidence of the disease is also higher among persons living in the temperate zone.

Several theories have been suggested, but the cause of rheumatoid arthritis has not been identified. Immunological changes occur that cause destructive changes in the synovial tissues. The rheumatoid factor, an antibody that is present in the disease, plays a role in perpetuating inflammation through reaction with the body's immunoglobulins.

Signs and symptoms

Rheumatoid arthritis is usually polyarticular and involves the small joints of the hands and feet. The involvement is symmetrical, and the joints ache with motion and with rest. Motion is limited by pain and stiffness. The onset of the disease is generally insidious, but acute onset can occur. The latter has a better prognosis. The cardinal signs of inflammation, warmth, redness, swelling, and tenderness also differentiate the disease from osteo-arthritis.

The appearance of signs and symptoms is characterized by early morning stiffness that persists for an hour or more. Pain is more pronounced after exercise and progresses during the day. The small joints of the hands, feet, and wrists are particularly vulnerable. In advanced disease, classic deformities appear: subcutaneous nodules around elbows and fingers, partial dislocations of the cervical spine, flexion contracture with ankylosing of the wrists and fingers, and flexion contractures of the hips and knees. Systemic complaints of fatigue, malaise, fever, and weight loss may be present.

The American Rheumatism Association (1973) has established the following 11 criteria for diagnosing rheumatoid arthritis:

1. Morning stiffness
2. Pain on motion or tenderness in at least one joint
3. Swelling (soft tissue thickening or fluid—not bony overgrowth) in at least one joint continuously for 6 weeks or more
4. Swelling of at least one other joint
5. Symmetrical joint swelling
6. Subcutaneous nodules
7. X-ray changes typical of rheumatoid arthritis
8. Positive rheumatoid factor
9. Poor mucin precipitate from synovial fluid
10. Characteristic histological changes in synovial fluid
11. Characteristic histological changes in nodules

These symptoms must be present for 6 weeks to make a diagnosis. The presence of seven symptoms is classified as classic disease, five symptoms as definite, and three as possible.

Management

A variety of modalities of therapy are used in the management of rheumatoid arthritis, but this chapter will be limited to management with medication. The aim of drug therapy is to relieve pain and inflammation and to arrest the disease. Drug management for the various types of arthritic diseases is achieved with a wide variety of medications. Those included in this section are nonsteroidal antiinflammatory agents, phenylbutazone, indomethacin, gold salts, penicillamine, and hydroxychloroquine.

Nonsteroidal antiinflammatory agents

The nonsteroidal antiinflammatory drugs (NSAID) inhibit prostaglandin synthesis, and this inhibition probably produces antirheumatic activity by decreasing the prostaglandin level in arthritic joints. NSAID (Table 4), including aspirin but excluding indomethacin and phenylbutazone, are discussed as a group because of the common side effects that occur in any age population. Health professionals should be alert to these side effects that appear in older adults, because they are frequently thought to be the classic complaints of old age. Specific information relevant to the individual drugs will be in the section that follows.

Common side effects of aspirin and other NSAID

Asthmalike symptoms. Bronchial spasm, running nose, and difficult breathing are manifestations of an allergic response to aspirin. These symptoms may be induced by other NSAID that contain aspirin. Accurate allergy histories are necessary, and test doses of aspirin with close monitoring are recommended when an allergy is suspected.

CNS symptoms. Dementia, psychosis, depression, Parkinson's tremors, fatigue, and headache may occur with several NSAID. These problems are relatively rare, but because of their severity in older adults, health professionals, patients, and families must be on the alert for them.

Renal toxicity. Transient elevations in blood urea nitrogen and serum creatinine may occur early in the course of therapy with aspirin and NSAID. Decreased renal function is a particular problem with the older population.

Edema and weight gain. Water retention with or without sodium retention may be caused by salicylates and other NSAID. The fluid retention may not be readily responsive to diuretics.

Hepatitis. Anorexia, lethargy, dark urine, and jaundice may occur during therapy.

Gastrointestinal irritation. The aspirin component of NSAID has a corrosive effect on stomach tissue. Symptoms that may occur range from gastric upset to gastric bleeding with the associated coffee-ground emesis and tarry stools or stools mixed with bright red blood. The problem is exaggerated with the ingestion of alcohol.

Phenylbutazone

Drug action. The antiinflammatory effects of phenylbutazone are similar to those of the salicylates. Mild uricosuric effects are seen at doses of approximately 600 mg/day. Antipyretic and analgesic effects are also present, but toxicity limits the drug's usefulness in these areas.

Drug	Dosage
Phenylbutazone	Acute gouty arthritis: 400 mg as an initial dose, then 100 mg every 4 hours for approximately 4 days or until the desired outcome is achieved; therapy is not to exceed 7 days.
	Rheumatoid arthritis and other rheumatic diseases: 100 to 200 mg three times daily as an initial dose, then 100 to 200 mg one to four times daily as a maintenance dose.

Proper use and precautions
1. Medication is to be taken before or after meals or with a full glass of milk to minimize gastric irritation.
2. Alcohol and aspirin are to be avoided, because they increase the possibility of gastric irritation.
3. Improvement in the condition should occur within 3 to 4 days.
4. The medication should be used with caution for older adults with impaired cardiac, renal, and liver function; edema; hypertension; gastrointestinal irritation or ulceration; and blood dyscrasias.
5. Drug interactions may occur with anticoagulants (potentiate hypoprothrombinemic effects), digitoxin (serum levels may be decreased), hypoglycemics (effects may be potentiated), phenytoin (may increase half-life with danger of phenytoin toxicity), and salicylates (inhibit uricosuric effect).
6. Side effects especially prominent in the elderly and persons with medical conditions previously identified include hearing loss, bloody stools or urine, urination problems, difficulty in breathing, indigestion or stomach pain, eye pain or visual changes, skin rash, sore throat or fever, edema, ulcers or white spots in mouth, unusual bleeding or bruising, unusual fatigue, unusual weight gain, and signs of jaundice.
7. Because of drowsiness or other symptoms of decreasing alertness, the patient should be cautioned to avoid driving or operating mechanical household equipment or appliances.
8. Monitoring includes regular physician visits, complete blood count, and urinalysis.

Indomethacin

Drug action. The analgesic, antipyretic actions of indomethacin reduce pain, swelling, and joint tenderness in moderate to severe rheumatoid and degenerative disorders.

TABLE 4. Nonsteroidal antiinflammatory drugs used in rheumatic diseases

Drug	Dose	Administration	Drug interactions	Caution with medical problems	Other monitoring
Acetylsalicylic acid (aspirin)	3.6-5.4 gm daily in divided doses	With food or full glass of water or milk	Alcohol, other antiinflammatory agents, urinary acidifiers or alkalizers, oral anticoagulants, oral hypoglycemics, probenecid, methotrexate.	Peptic ulcer, hemophilia, other bleeding problems, asthma, allergy, nasal polyps, gout, anemia, Hodgkin's disease, renal and hepatic function impairment.	Serum salicylate levels.
Ibuprofen	400 mg q.4h.	With meals or milk	Alcohol, other antiinflammatory agents, anticoagulants, previous reactions to aspirin.	Bleeding problems, peptic ulcers.	Maximum effectiveness may take 1-2 wk.
Sulindac	150-200 mg b.i.d.	With meals or milk	Alcohol, other antiinflammatory agents, previous reactions to aspirin, probenecid.	Bleeding problems, nasal polyps, peptic ulcers; patients with impaired renal function may require lower doses.	Effect may take 2-3 wk.

Drug	Dose	Administration	Precautions	Adverse effects	Onset
Fenoprofen	300-600 mg q.i.d.	30 min before or 2 hr after meals	Alcohol, other antiinflammatory agents, anticoagulants, previous reactions to aspirin.	Bleeding problems, peptic ulcers.	Effect may take 2-3 wk.
Naproxen	250 mg b.i.d.	With meals or milk	Alcohol, other antiinflammatory agents, anticoagulants, previous reactions to aspirin.	Bleeding problems, peptic ulcers; patients with impaired renal or cranial nerve function may require lower doses.	Effect may take 2-3 wk.
Tolmetin	0.6-1.8 gm daily in divided doses	With meals, milk, or antacids (except sodium bicarbonate)	Alcohol, other antiinflammatory agents, anticoagulants, previous reactions to aspirin; sodium bicarbonate may enhance excretion.	Bleeding problems, peptic ulcers; patients with impaired renal function may require lower doses.	Improvement comes within a few days to 1 wk.
Piroxicam	20 mg daily	Morning or night	Aspirin decreases plasma levels.	Bleeding problems, peptic ulcers.	Therapeutic effects begin early and increase for several weeks.

Drug	Dosage
Indomethacin	Antigout: Initially 100 mg, then 50 mg three times daily until pain is reduced, with a rapid decrease in dosage until discontinued.
	Antipyretic: 25 to 50 mg three to four times daily.
	Antirheumatic: Initially 25 to 50 mg two to four times daily with dose increased to a maximum of 200 mg daily. Also available in 75 mg sustained-release dosage form for once- or twice-a-day dosing.

Proper use and precautions

1. Medication is to be taken after meals or with food or milk to decrease gastric irritation.
2. Before the patient has any type of surgery, the physician or dentist should be informed about this drug.
3. Alcohol and aspirin should be avoided, because they increase the possibility of gastric irritation.
4. Effects of medication may not be observed until 2 to 4 weeks after the initiation of therapy.
5. Geriatric patients require careful monitoring, because they are particularly susceptible to adverse reactions.
6. The medication should be used with caution for older adults with gastrointestinal lesions, bleeding problems, previous reactions to aspirin or aspirin-containing medications, and renal or hepatic impairment.
7. Drug interactions may occur with alcohol or antiinflammatory drugs (increase ulcerogenic effects), anticoagulants (potential for development of gastrointestinal ulceration increases danger of hemorrhage), and probenecid (causes a rise in the serum levels of indomethacin, which can increase effectiveness as well as toxicity danger).
8. Side effects to which older adults are especially vulnerable include nausea, vomiting, or other forms of gastric distress, including bloody or tarry stools; ringing in the ears or other hearing problems; visual or mental changes; dyspnea or other symptoms of respiratory distress; edema or unexplained weight gain; skin rashes, sore throat, or fever; unusual bleeding or bruising; and signs of jaundice.
9. Because dizziness may occur, the patient should be cautioned to avoid driving or using mechanical household equipment or appliances.
10. Monitoring includes regular physician visits, blood cell counts, and stool examinations for occult blood and ophthalmoscopic examination if the patient is receiving prolonged therapy.

Remission-inducing agents

Gold salts. Gold salts may be the drug of choice when one or more of the following conditions exists: test result for the rheumatoid factor is seropositive; the disease is active, progressive, and erosive; NSAID have proven ineffective; or there is a previous history of peptic ulcers. Because of the potential side effects, patients are encouraged to discuss these problems in detail with the rheumatologist.

Drug action. Gold salts are reported to decrease synovial inflammation and retard cartilage and bone destruction.

Drug	Dosage
Gold sodium thiomalate	Intramuscular only. Initial: 10 mg first week, 25 mg second week, then 25 to 50 mg weekly until desired response or toxicity occurs, up to a maximum total dose of 1 gm. Maintenance: 25 to 50 mg every 2 weeks for 2 to 20 weeks; then 25 to 50 mg every 3 to 4 weeks.
Aurothioglucose suspension	Intramuscular only. Initial: 10 mg first week, 25 mg second and third weeks, then 50 mg weekly until a total dose of 800 to 1000 mg has been given. Maintenance: 25 to 50 mg every 3 to 4 weeks.
Auranofin	Oral: 1 to 6 mg/day (Bernhard, 1982).

Proper use and precautions
1. The patient should be lying down when the intramuscular form is administered and remain in this position for 10 to 15 minutes because of possible reactions.
2. Symptoms that may appear immediately following administration include dizziness, feeling faint, facial flushing, nausea or vomiting, and unusual perspiration or weakness.
3. Drug interactions are possible with dermatitis-producing medications.
4. Exposure to sunlight should be minimized.
5. The medication should be used with caution for persons with active renal disease, previous sensitivity to heavy metals, blood dyscrasias, Sjögren's syndrome in rheumatoid arthritis and systemic lupus erythematosus, hypertension or other cardiovascular problems, liver disease, and skin diseases.
6. Side effects may appear immediately following administration or months after the drug was administered. Side effects that should be reported immediately include irritation and soreness of tongue or gums with possible ulceration, metallic taste in mouth, skin rash, or

itching. Long-term side effects include unusual fatigue, bruising or bleeding, visual problems, yellowish or greyish blue skin discoloration, and unusual sensations in hands or feet.

7. Monitoring includes regular physician visits, complete blood counts including platelets, and urinalysis.

Penicillamine. Penicillamine is used for rheumatoid arthritis, Wilson's disease, lead poisoning, and the prevention of kidney stones. The discussion in this section is limited to its use for rheumatoid arthritis.

Drug action. Penicillamine suppresses rheumatoid disease activity by an unknown mechanism of action.

Drug	Dosage
Penicillamine capsules Penicillamine tablets	Initial: 125 to 250 mg daily as a single dose; the dose is increased as necessary by adding 125 to 250 mg daily at 1 to 3 month intervals up to 1.5 gm daily.

Proper use and precautions

1. Dosages up to 500 mg/day should be given in a single dose.
2. Medication should be taken on an empty stomach at least 1 hour before meals and at least 1 hour apart from any other medications, food, or milk to ensure maximum absorption and reduce the possibility of inactivation by metal binding.
3. Response to therapy may not appear for 2 to 3 months.
4. Medications containing iron and some vitamins should not be taken within 2 hours of the time this medication is taken. Iron may decrease the effects of penicillamine.
5. This medication must be taken precisely as directed and not discontinued without consultation with the physician. Stopping and restarting the medication may increase the possibility of sensitivity.
6. The physician or dentist should be informed about this drug before any surgical procedure because of the effects on collagen and elastin.
7. Supplemental pyridoxine should be given during therapy, because penicillamine increases the requirement for this vitamin.
8. This medication is contraindicated for persons with penicillin allergies or with a history of renal disease.
9. Penicillamine should not be used for patients receiving gold therapy, antimalarial or cytotoxic drugs, or phenylbutazone.
10. Multiple side effects may occur with this medication. Those occurring most frequently and requiring medical attention include fever, joint pain, skin rashes, hives, itching, enlarged lymph nodes, bloody or cloudy urine, sore throat and fever, unusual bleeding or bruising, and unusual fatigue. Gastrointestinal problems of anorexia, nausea, and vomiting may also occur. The patient should be urged to discuss with

the physician the possibility of additional serious but rarer side effects.

11. Monitoring includes regular visits to the physician; complete blood count, including white blood cell, hemoglobin, differential, and platelets; hepatic function tests; and urinalysis for protein.

Hydroxychloroquine. Hydroxychloroquine is an antimalarial drug used in arthritic patients who have been unresponsive to more conservative forms of therapy. Many months of therapy may be needed for remission to occur. This drug is used in other types of therapy, but our discussion pertains only to rheumatoid arthritis.

Drug action. Mechanism of antiinflammatory action is unknown.

Drug	Dosage
Hydroxychloroquine sulfate tablets	Initial: 400 to 600 mg daily until the desired response is reached.
	Maintenance: 200 to 400 mg daily.

Proper use and precautions

1. Medication should be taken with meals or milk to minimize gastric irritation.
2. Concurrent use of hydroxychloroquine with phenylbutazone and gold salts increases the possibility of skin reactions.
3. The medication should be used with caution for patients who have severe blood, gastric, and neurological disorders and for those who have retinal field changes.
4. Because of the retinal changes that can occur with long-term therapy, an eye examination by an ophthalmologist before the start of therapy is essential. The elderly are especially susceptible to visual changes.
5. Side effects include gastrointestinal disturbances; blurred vision; bleaching of hair or hair loss; blue-black changes of skin, nails, and oral mucous membrane; skin rash or itching; sore throat and fever; bruising and unusual bleeding; muscle weakness; and tinnitus.
6. Acidification of the urine will hasten elimination of the drug in patients having overdosage or sensitivity reactions.
7. Monitoring includes regular visits to the physician, visual changes, ophthalmoscopic examination every 6 months and following therapy, and complete blood count.

GOUT

Gout is the physical manifestation of a metabolic disorder that is characterized by hyperuricemia, or abnormally high levels of uric acid in the blood.

The incidence of the disease increases with age. Before the age of 50, men are more commonly affected, but after 50 the incidence in women increases. Gout and hyperuricemia are not synonymous terms. Not all persons with hyperuricemia develop gout. There does seem to be a correlation among the level of the serum uric acid, duration of hyperuricemia, manifestations of acute gout, appearance of tophi, and the complication of renal stones.

Drugs known to induce the hyperuricemia associated with gout include the thiazide diuretics, alcohol, levodopa, nicotinic acid, ethambutol, and the contrast dye agents used in diagnostic studies.

Signs and symptoms

Although any joint may be involved, the most commonly involved joint is the great toe. The involvement, sudden in onset, produces excruciating pain, with a reddened, swollen joint and surrounding tissues. The foot is extremely sensitive to any pressure, including the weight of bed linens. When gout is poorly controlled, small nodules called tophi, containing uric acid crystals, may appear on the ears, elbows, and hands. Uric acid crystals are present in the substance aspirated from the joint and tophi. Laboratory tests will indicate elevated serum uric acid, sedimentation rate, and white blood cells.

Management

The aim of therapy for an acute attack of gout is to reduce the severity of the pain and quickly terminate the acute inflammatory process. The drug of choice in acute undiagnosed but suspected gout is colchicine. The NSAID, indomethacin, and phenylbutazone are also effective in the management of acute gouty arthritis.

Three types of drugs are used in the treatment of acute or chronic gout: (1) drugs to control the acute inflammatory process—colchicine, indomethacin, and phenylbutazone; (2) drugs to increase the excretion of uric acid from the kidneys—probenecid and sulfinpyrazone; and (3) drugs to reduce the production of uric acid—allopurinol. Drugs included in the discussion of gout are colchicine and allopurinol. Indomethacin and phenylbutazone have been previously discussed in the management of arthritis.

Antigout agents
Colchicine

Drug action. Colchicine stops the chain reaction that occurs when urate crystals form in the joint. The drug keeps the polymorphonuclear cells from migrating into the joints and attempting to engulf the foreign bodies. It also prevents the leukocytes that enter the joint from releasing lactic acid and lysosomal enzymes. No additional crystals can precipitate in the joint fluid, and the possibility of joint damage decreases.

Drug	Dosage
Colchicine	Prophylactic: 0.5 to 0.65 mg one to three times daily. Therapeutic: 0.5 mg to 1.3 mg initially, then 0.5 mg to 0.65 mg every 1 to 2 hours or 1 to 1.3 mg every 2 hours until pain is relieved or until nausea, vomiting, or diarrhea occurs.

Proper use and precautions
1. If colchicine is taken only when an acute attack occurs, it must be taken in the prescribed dose at the first sign of the attack. The medication should be discontinued as soon as the pain ceases or at the first sign of nausea, vomiting, stomach pain, or diarrhea.
2. If colchicine is taken regularly to prevent gout, in the event of an acute attack an increased dose as prescribed by the physician is taken. Precautions as indicated in the preceding paragraph are applicable. The previous dose as prescribed by the physician is then resumed.
3. The dosage for geriatric patients who have renal or cardiac problems must be carefully monitored, because they are more susceptible to toxicity.
4. Alcohol must be avoided, because it may decrease the effects of colchicine.
5. The most common side effects are diarrhea, nausea, vomiting, and stomach pain, which indicate that the medication must be discontinued. If the symptoms persist, the physician should be notified. Other problems with long-term use include numbness, tingling, pain or weakness of the hands or feet, skin rash, sore throat or fever, unusual bleeding or bruising, and unusual weakness or fatigue.
6. Monitoring includes complete blood counts at regular intervals and regular physician visits.

Allopurinol

Drug action. Allopurinol lowers serum levels of uric acid by interfering with the formation of uric acid rather than increasing its urinary excretion. Because of the lower amounts of uric acid in the urine, patients are less likely to develop renal stones.

Drug	Dosage
Allopurinol	100 to 200 mg two to three times daily or 300 mg as a single daily dose. To prevent acute gout attacks, an initial dose of 100 mg may be increased by 100 mg weekly until a serum uric acid level of 6 mg/dl or less is reached.

Proper use and precautions
1. Medication should be taken with meals to minimize gastrointestinal irritation.
2. Since allopurinol may increase the incidence of acute gouty arthritis early in therapy, prophylactic doses of colchicine are frequently given.
3. Patients receiving concurrent uricosuric agents should drink at least 2.5 to 3 L of liquids daily to maintain a neutral or slightly acid urine and thereby reduce the risk of xanthine calculi formations and precipitation of urates.
4. The drug should be given with caution to older adults with impaired renal function.
5. Drug interactions may occur with ampicillin (increased possibility of skin rash), alcohol, thiazide and other diuretics (increase in serum uric acid level), anticoagulants (anticoagulant effect may be potentiated), azathioprine or mercaptopurine (effects may be potentiated), and urinary acidifiers including vitamin C (increased possibility of renal stone formation).
6. Side effects include skin rash and pruritis, unusual sensations or weakness in hands or feet, unusual bruising or bleeding, unusual weakness, and signs of jaundice.
7. Because drowsiness may occur, the patient should be cautioned about driving a car or operating household mechanical equipment or appliances.
8. Monitoring includes regular physician visits, complete blood count, hepatic and renal function tests, and serum uric acid levels.

OSTEOPOROSIS

Osteoporosis is presumed to develop from an imbalance over a long time between bone resorption and formation. The bones become more porous, weaker, brittle, and susceptible to fracture. Because the incidence of the disease shows a striking increase among older women, it is frequently referred to as senile or postmenopausal osteoporosis. In the late midlife years the incidence ratio of women to men is 2:1, but by the eighth decade there is no difference between sexes. In women over 65 the prevalence has been reported to range between 30% and 80% (Spencer and Lender, 1979).

Many etiological factors have been considered to have a role in the development of osteoporosis. A certain amount of osteoporosis occurs as part of the normal aging process, possibly because of lower levels of sex hormones. It has been demonstrated that estrogen therapy increases calcium absorption in postmenopausal women. Inactivity, which becomes increasingly more common in old people, is responsible for bone loss. The normal weight-bearing position places stress on the long bones, thereby stimulating bone formation. Improper nutritional intake throughout life has an effect on the maintenance of a healthy skeletal system. The nutrients that help promote structural integrity include calcium, phosphorus, protein, and vitamins C and D. A lack or imbalance of these nutrients can contribute to the development of osteoporosis. White women of small stature are also more prone to develop the disease. Chronic illnesses in which secondary osteoporosis can occur include hyperthyroidism, hyperparathyroidism, Cushing's syndrome, chronic uremia, alcoholism, malabsorption syndromes, and a postgastrectomy state. The wide variety of etiological factors that contribute to the development of osteoporosis is an indication of the difficulty in defining effective therapy.

Signs and symptoms

The insidious onset and lack of symptoms for prolonged periods are responsible for a delay in diagnosis. Lumbar or midthoracic pain caused by collapse and fracture of the vertebrae may be the first symptom. This back pain and further collapse may be aggravated by any movement, such as sneezing, brushing the teeth, or opening a window. Unfortunately, the first symptom may be the severe pain associated with the fracture of the neck of the femur, which is a very vulnerable site. Several other findings that may indicate this condition include kyphosis, decrease in lordotic curve, limitation of motion, and decrease in height.

Management

If the causes of osteoporosis were more clearly defined, a management program focusing on the prevention of bone resorption and the promotion of bone formation could be planned. However, with the present knowledge of the disease, the goals are directed to decreasing progression of the disease, preventing complications, and promoting comfort.

Nutritional counseling is an essential part of therapy. The practitioner needs to work with the patient in planning a diet rich in calcium, vitamin D, and protein. Good food sources of calcium include milk and other dairy products, eggs, broccoli, canned fish, nuts, and greens.

To promote comfort for patients with osteoporosis, the practitioner can recommend a moderate program of weight-bearing and muscle-setting exercises. Analgesics must be used judiciously. Supportive devices such as corsets and belts are helpful in relieving pain but are often too cumbersome to wear.

Warm packs, heating pads, and gentle massage may be useful in relieving the pain and discomfort in specific body areas.

Specific drug therapy is designed to correct the two assumed defects in osteoporosis, decreasing bone resorption and increasing bone formation. Spencer and Lender (1979) indicate that estrogens and calcitonin fall into the first category, whereas calcium supplements and fluoride probably fit into both categories.

To achieve adequate calcium levels, supplements in minimum doses of 1 gm daily are recommended. High doses of calcium convert the calcium balance in the older person from negative to positive, but recalcification of the bones is questionable. Long-term fluoride therapy has been used to improve the structure of the skeletal system, and some research indicates improvement. Fractures have occurred less frequently and bone pain is less severe in selective patients receiving fluoride.

Estrogens produce symptomatic relief and temporarily diminish progression of the disease in most patients by decreasing urinary calcium excretion and improving calcium balance, and some evidence indicates a decreased rate of bone resorption. Gordon and Vaughan (1977) report success in the prevention of bone loss with another hormone, porcine calcitonin. The treatment of osteoporosis with drugs remains controversial, because results do not indicate an increase in bone density.

REFERENCES

American Rheumatism Association: Primer on rheumatic diseases, ed. 7, New York, 1973, The Foundation.
Bernhard, G.C.: Auranofin therapy in rheumatoid arthritis, J. Lab. Clin. Med. **100**:167, 1982.
Gordon, G., and Vaughan, C.: The role of estrogens in osteoporosis, Geriatrics **32**:42, 1977.
Spencer, H., and Lender, M.: The skeletal system. In Rossman, I., editor: Clinical geriatrics, Philadelphia, 1979, J.B. Lippincott Co.

SUGGESTED READINGS

Bienenstock, H., and Fernando, K.: Arthritis in the elderly: an overview, Med. Clin. North Am. **60**:1173, 1976.
Brewerton, D.: Rheumatic disorders. In Rossman, I., editor: Clinical geriatrics, Philadelphia, 1979, J.B. Lippincott Co.
Jowsey, J.: Osteoporosis: dealing with a crippling bone disease of the elderly, Geriatrics **32**:41, 1977.
Richards, M.: Osteoporosis, Geriatr. Nurs. **3**:98, 1982.
Wheeler, M.: Osteoporosis, Med. Clin. North Am. **69**:1213, 1976.

10

MANAGEMENT OF SELECTED ENDOCRINE PROBLEMS

The major endocrine problem encountered by older persons is diabetes mellitus. The increasing incidence of diabetes in the elderly population, the serious complications that occur, and the responsibility for self-management have an impact on the role of the practitioner. Thyroid diseases and their therapy are also included in this chapter.

DIABETES MELLITUS

The increased incidence of diabetes in the older population requires health practitioners to be alert to the needs of elderly persons in whom diabetes has been identified and to situations in which symptoms may indicate the possibility of the illness. The prevalence of this disorder, which shows a distinct increase after the age of 50, will continue to rise as more people live to old age. However, after 85 years the incidence of newly diagnosed diabetes begins to fall.

The diagnosis of diabetes in older adults becomes problematic, because decreased glucose tolerance, which is also considered a normal change associated with the aging process, can be affected by inactivity, poor nutrition or severe carbohydrate restriction, stressful illnesses, and other problems associated with the endocrine system. Certain drugs taken by older persons that may also decrease glucose tolerance include thiazides, furosemide, levodopa, and phenytoin.

If possible, factors affecting glucose tolerance should be corrected and additional glucose tolerance tests performed before making a diagnosis of diabetes. The glucose tolerance test is interpreted by using age-related gradients. Eliopoulous (1978) suggests that for every 10 years, beginning at age 55, 10 mg of glucose be added to the standard value at the first, second, and third hours. Andres and associates (1967) published a nomogram that is useful for screening.

Because of the availability of home urine testing methods, mention should be made of the renal threshold for glucose, which rises as part of the aging process. An older person may be hyperglycemic and have no indication of glycosuria. Fasting blood glucose levels may also be misleading, because they may not reveal an elevation, but postprandial tests will indicate hyperglycemia.

Signs and symptoms

Older persons may not develop polydipsia, polyuria, and polyphagia, the classic signs of diabetes that are associated with younger persons. The higher renal threshold permits the accumulation of higher levels of glucose. In younger persons, thirst and excessive urination occur when the kidneys excrete extra fluid. However, with older persons these symptoms may not occur, since the glucose is not excreted until it reaches higher levels.

The older adult may seek health care because of the complications of diabetes rather than because of the usual clinical manifestations. Diabetes may have been present for years without any obvious indication of its presence. During this period, levels of glucose accumulate and are partially responsible for the skin disorders; peripheral and visceral neuropathies; and renal, eye, and other complications. The prevalence of these complications is directly related to the degree and duration of hyperglycemia.

Another complication that may be the first indication of diabetes is hyperosmolar nonketotic coma, which is a syndrome that may occur in older persons who are not known to be diabetic and in persons who may be controlled with diet or oral hypoglycemic agents. Blood glucose rises to extremely high levels, and the accompanying glycosuria leads to polyuria and dehydration. Water intake increases but is insufficient to prevent the increase in osmolarity that accompanies fluid loss and increasing blood glucose. With the increasing osmolarity, dehydration occurs, and the person may also be confused or comatose. Because the situation is life threatening, immediate intensive treatment is essential.

Management

An assessment of the effect that this chronic illness may have on the person's life-style is imperative before establishing therapeutic goals. Present eating patterns need to be assessed before a rigid diet is prescribed, because it is possible that some favorite foods may be continued. A thorough health assessment and communication of the results to health team members can contribute to a realistic plan of care. Diabetes in the older patient can frequently be controlled with diet alone, but sometimes the addition of an oral hypoglycemic agent or insulin is necessary.

Drug therapy and other interventions in the control of diabetes are procedures that may be problematic for the older person. Many of these problems partially relate to the changes associated with aging. Urine testing is a relatively simple procedure and is recommended unless the renal glucose threshold is very high. In situations in which the threshold is high, a comparison of urine with simultaneous blood glucose can be done. This information will offer some validity to the urine testing, if the results are correctly interpreted.

Another important factor in urine testing is the use of a second voided specimen, which gives an indication of the amount of glucose in the body at the time of testing. To obtain this specimen the person must completely empty the bladder and then void again for the second specimen. Because of the loss of muscle tone in the aging bladder, the person may be unable to completely empty the bladder. The results may then present an inaccurate picture, and if intervention is based on these values, problems may occur. Therefore, if the inability of the person to empty the bladder completely is confirmed by catheterization, other means of monitoring should be explored (Hayter, 1981).

The first voided specimen is a screening tool that is recommended by Guthrie and Guthrie (1982). Although this specimen does not identify the time of the glucose spillage, it does indicate the spillage within 4 to 6 hours before voiding. The first voided specimen before each meal and at bedtime offers reliable information. If the specimen is positive, spot specimens (second voided) can be taken at specified times to determine the more precise time of the spillage. In this method the first voided specimen is the screening tool and the second voided specimen the more definitive test. Because of the difficulty in fully emptying the bladder, the first voided specimen may be preferred.

Interpreting the results of the urine test may be difficult for the older person, since color vision may be altered because of the yellowing of the lens that accompanies aging. The discoloration of the lens makes it difficult to interpret the short wavelength colors of blue, green, and violet. This change in color perception may result in inaccuracies when the person is discriminating the blues and greens required in testing urine.

Older persons may also be taking over-the-counter and prescribed drugs that can affect the outcome of urine testing for glucose and ketones. Examples of drugs that may affect the outcome of urine testing for glucose and ketones are listed in Table 5. Because some urine testing methods are reported in pluses and some in percentage, the need for conversion from one

TABLE 5. Drugs that may affect the outcome of urine testing for glucose and ketones

	Clinitest	Clinistix	Tes-tape	Ketostix	Acetest
Ascorbic acid	False-positive	False-negative	False-negative		
Cephalosporins	False-positive				
Chloramphenicol	False-positive				
Levodopa	False-positive	False-negative	False-negative	False-positive	False-positive
Metaxalone	False-positive				
Methyldopa	False-positive		False-negative		
Nalidixic acid	False-positive				
Paraldehyde and ethanol					False-positive
Phenazopyridine		False-negative	False-negative or positive	False-positive	
Probenecid	False-positive				
Salicylates (moderate to high doses)	False-positive	False-negative	False-negative	False-positive	False-positive
Sulfonamides	False-positive				
Tetracyclines	False-positive	False-negative (parenteral)			

Modified from Lundin, D.: Am. J. Nurs. **78**:879, 1978.

method to another should be carefully evaluated to determine the patient's comprehension before a change is made (Lundin, 1978).

The introduction of home blood glucose monitoring systems provides a more accurate indication of blood glucose at a given time. The use of one of the home systems has the following advantages: (1) results can be used to make daily adjustments in insulin dosage, diet, and activity levels, and (2) normalization of blood glucose levels can prevent or delay the onset or progression of long-term complications of diabetes. The use of a home monitoring system is recommended for type I (insulin-dependent types) diabetes, and the use with type II (non-insulin-dependent types) diabetes may be recommended for better control. The expense of the various systems available and the follow-through demands must be thoroughly discussed with the patient. Older adults using one of the home systems can readily be taught how to alter insulin dosage, food, and activity according to the readings on the meter.

Impairment of visual acuity because of multiple eye changes can interfere with the measurement of insulin. The availability of syringes with colored plungers and other devices for persons with visual impairment is recommended. The reader is directed to a valuable resource prepared by the National Diabetes Information Clearing House, *Diabetes and Aging*. This publication suggests resources for professionals and consumers that will help promote improved self-management by older diabetic patients.

The emotional reaction of the newly diagnosed older diabetic patient to this illness is unpredictable. Having lived at a time when the serious effects of diabetes and its complications were common, the patient may be depressed or angry. Feelings that life may be shortened and life-style restricted may occur. Concern about the expense of medication and monitoring materials may also limit compliance. The amount of new information to be learned to manage health problems and coping with these changes contribute to a sense of inadequacy. All these factors need to be assessed before planning a teaching program. Every diabetic patient has a right to learn about the disease, its effect on life-style, and the various aspects of control. Whether the disease is controlled by diet alone, with the addition of an oral hypoglycemic agent, or with insulin, the person must learn how to live with a chronic illness managed by medications, diet, and exercise. Principles of teaching older adults may be found in Chapter 7.

Oral hypoglycemic agents

The sulfonylureas are used for patients with type II, non-insulin-dependent diabetes mellitus, who have pancreatic insulin reserves.

TABLE 6. Dosage and duration of action of sulfonylureas

Drug name	Action in hours		Usual dose	Maximum dose
	Onset	Duration		
Sulfonylureas				
Tolbutamide	½	6-12	1000 mg daily in 2-3 doses	2000 mg daily
Chlorpropamide	1	60	250 mg daily	750-1000 mg daily
Acetohexamide	½	12-24	500 mg daily in 2 doses	1500 mg daily
Tolazamide	4-6	12-24	250 mg daily	750-1000 mg daily

Sulfonylureas

Drug action. Sulfonylureas stimulate insulin secretion from the pancreatic beta cells. Enhancement of glucose-induced insulin is a major factor in improved carbohydrate metabolism. The compounds are primarily metabolized in the liver to active metabolites and are then excreted by the liver at varying rates; the rate of excretion determines the length of action (Table 6).

Proper use and precautions
1. For geriatric patients with renal insufficiency, the dose should be initiated at a lower level and increased very slowly.
2. The importance of eating a prescribed diet to aid in the control of diabetes must be emphasized.
3. Medication is to be taken exactly as prescribed, at the same time each day.
4. Alcohol must be avoided, because it may cause abdominal pain, nausea, vomiting, headache, and flushing of the face and skin. Alcohol may also induce hypoglycemia.
5. Before the patient has any type of surgery, the physician or dentist should be informed about the medication.
6. No additional medications, including over-the-counter drugs, should be taken unless prescribed by a physician who knows that the person is taking a sulfonylurea.
7. The drug may produce hypoglycemia, which is characterized by anxiety, chills, perspiration, pallor, drowsiness, headache, nausea, nervousness, trembling, rapid pulse, and weakness. However, the older person may not exhibit the classic symptoms but may show episodes of bizarre behavior, slurred speech, disorientation, and confusion.

8. Caution should be used in sun exposure, because the medication may increase sensitivity to direct sunlight.
9. Drug interactions may occur with alcohol, guanethidine, insulin, MAO inhibitors, phenylbutazone, probenecid, sulfonamides, salicylates (may increase hypoglycemic effect), coumarin-type anticoagulants (may affect plasma levels of both drugs), propranolol (may mask symptoms of hypoglycemia), corticosteroids, phenytoin, thiazide diuretics, or thyroid hormones (may increase blood glucose levels).
10. Among the side effects that may occur are hypoglycemic reaction, dark urine, fatigue, fever or sore throat, skin itching or rash, pale stools, unusual bleeding or bruising, yellowing of skin or eyes, anorexia, heartburn, stomach discomfort, nausea, vomiting, diarrhea, and increased sensitivity to direct sunlight.
11. Monitoring includes regular visits to physician or other health practitioner, blood glucose determination, urine glucose tests, and urine ketone tests.
12. Specific comments regarding chlorpropamide:

   - Low doses are recommended, and it should be used with caution for older patients, who are more sensitive to its effects because of altered excretion and metabolism.
   - Additional side effects that may occur include drowsiness; muscle cramps; seizures; edema of face, hands, and ankles; fatigue; and weakness.
   - Its prolonged but unpredictable half-life indicates that several weeks may be required for complete elimination from the body.
   - Prolonged hypoglycemic reactions require close supervision for 3 to 5 days.

Insulin. Diabetes in older adults may also be controlled by insulin in addition to diet. Table 7 should be helpful to the practitioner when counseling patients regarding insulin administration.

Proper use and precautions
1. Insulin must be kept in balance with food intake and exercise. Patients should be taught the variables for dosage adjustment.
2. Appropriate methods of insulin administration, including rotation of sites and mixing insulin, and information about the various types of insulin should be part of a teaching program.
3. Monitoring urine and blood glucose provides a means of evaluating insulin therapy.
4. The bottle of insulin in use should be kept at room temperature, and other bottles should be stored in the refrigerator.
5. Bracelets that identify the patient as diabetic are recommended.
6. Drug interactions may occur. See Chapter 4.

TABLE 7. Comparison of insulin preparations

Insulin	Action in hours			Compatible mixed with
	Onset	Peak	Duration	
Rapid acting				
Insulin injection				
Insulin (regular)	½-1	2-4	6-8	All insulin preparations
Insulin, zinc suspension				
Semilente insulin	½-1	2-4	8-10	Lente preparations
Intermediate acting				
Isophane insulin suspension				
Isophane insulin (NPH)	1-2	6-8	12-14	Insulin injection
Insulin, zinc suspension				
Lente insulin	1-2	6-8	14-16	Insulin injection, semilente
Long acting				
Extended zinc insulin suspension				
Ultralente insulin	4-6	8-12	24-36	Insulin injection, semilente
Protamine zinc insulin suspension				
Protamine zinc insulin	4-6	18+	36-72	*Insulin injection

Adapted from Larner, J. In Goodman, L.S., and others, editors: The pharmacological basis of therapeutics, ed. 6, New York, 1980, Macmillan Publishing Co., Inc.; and from Guthrie, D.W., and Guthrie, R.A.: Nursing management of diabetes mellitus, ed. 2, St. Louis, 1982, The C.V. Mosby Co.

*When protamine zinc insulin (PZI) is mixed with regular insulin, the excess free protamine combines with the regular insulin to give varying durations of action. In proportions of 1:1, the duration is approximately equal to that of PZI alone. When the regular insulin exceeds PZI more than 2:1, the activity resembles that of a mixture of regular and NPH insulin.

7. Side effects that may occur include localized skin reactions, fluctuations in blood pressure and pulse rates, hunger, nausea, vomiting, lethargy, confusion, and diaphoresis.
8. Monitoring includes regular visits to a health-care professional, blood glucose determination, urinalysis for glucose and ketones, and observation for hyperglycemia and hypoglycemia.

HYPOTHYROIDISM

Hypothyroidism is primarily a disease of the aged that reaches its peak in the fifth, sixth, and seventh decades of life. After diabetes, it is the second most common endocrine disease of older adults. As with other thyroid diseases, hypothyroidism is most common in women, involving women five times more frequently than men. The changes that a person undergoes because of this deficiency are frequently attributed to old age, and as a result the diagnosis may be overlooked.

The disease may occur as a result of treatment for hyperthyroidism (surgery or administration of radioactive iodine), untreated chronic thyroiditis, Graves' disease, and the administration of drugs that may interfere with thyroid metabolism. Drugs known to be etiological factors include lithium, sulfonylureas, and occasionally phenylbutazone.

Signs and symptoms

The manifestations of hypothyroidism, which are also common complaints of older persons, include lethargy, apathy, intolerance to cold, constipation, impaired memory, and generally slowed responses. The hair becomes dry and lifeless, the skin is dry and thickened, the eyelids are puffy, the voice is husky and weak, and the tongue thickens. As the disease progresses, bradycardia, angina pectoris, weakness, and general myopathy occur. Because the illness is so gradual and insidious in its onset, the person may accept these changes as part of growing old, and unfortunately, the disease progresses.

Management

Following confirmation of hypothyroidism through thyroid function studies, treatment to replace thyroid hormone is instituted. Two types of thyroid hormone preparations are available: natural preparations derived from the thyroid glands of domesticated animals and synthetic compounds that have the advantage of not requiring standardization. Thyroid hormone USP and sodium levothyroxine are the drugs most frequently used to treat hypothyroidism in the elderly. Treatment is begun with small doses and increased at 2-week intervals until optimum effects are obtained.

Thyroid preparations
Thyroid

Drug action. Thyroid regulates the rate of metabolism in all body cells.

Drug	Dosage
Thyroid USP	Maintenance: 90 to 180 mg/day.
Sodium levothyroxine	Maintenance: 0.05 to 0.2 mg/day.

Proper use and precautions
1. Lower dosages with small increments may be required for elderly patients and persons with myxedema and cardiovascular disease.
2. Medication is to be taken exactly as prescribed.
3. Medication is not to be discontinued without consulting the physician, because this therapy may be a lifelong process. Older persons who have been on long-term therapy should be evaluated for correct dosage and the need for continued therapy.
4. Other medications, including over-the-counter drugs, are to be avoided unless prescribed by a physician.
5. For persons with some types of coronary artery disease, the medicine may induce chest pain or dyspnea on exertion. Therefore strenuous physical work and exercise should be avoided.
6. Before the patient has any type of surgery, the physician or dentist should be notified about this medication.
7. Drug interactions may occur with oral anticoagulants (thyroid may increase anticoagulant effects), antidiabetic agents, insulin (thyroid may increase blood glucose), cholestyramine (may decrease the effects of thyroid), phenytoin (may increase effects of thyroid), sympathomimetics, or tricyclic antidepressants (may increase effects of both medications).
8. Side effects that require immediate attention include chest pain, rapid or irregular heartbeat, shortness of breath, hives or skin rash, tremors, nervousness, insomnia, irritability, headaches, leg cramps, change in appetite, weight loss, vomiting, diarrhea, sensitivity to heat, fever, and unusual sweating; other side effects related to underdosage include dry puffy skin, coldness, sleepiness, unusual weight gain, listlessness, weakness, headache, muscle aches, and constipation.
9. Monitoring includes regular physician visits, thyroid function tests, electrocardiogram, regular recording of weight, and observation for

signs and symptoms of overdosage or underdosage (very significant with older persons and persons with cardiovascular disease because of sensitivity).

HYPERTHYROIDISM

Recent data suggest that as many as one third of thyrotoxic patients are over 60 years of age and that three fourths of this population have classic symptoms of thyroid hyperfunction (Davis, 1977). As with hypothyroidism, the symptoms are often interpreted as part of the aging process, not as thyroid dysfunction. Most older adults with this problem seek health care for significant diseases of other organ systems, and the thyroid problem may be ignored. The "other" disease may also trigger the onset of hyperthyroidism.

Signs and symptoms

The onset of hyperthyroidism in older persons is generally insidious and may present itself in an atypical manner. The patient may appear more apathetic, depressed, and lethargic than does a younger person with this problem. Other signs and symptoms include anorexia, weight loss, constipation, and insomnia. Cardiovascular findings in the older age group include cardiac arrhythmias, angina pectoris, congestive heart failure, and similar tachycardia found in other age groups. Exophthalmos is less common and less severe in older persons, with mild manifestations occurring in about 40% of the patients. The muscle weakness found in older persons becomes more profound, particularly in the quadriceps and deltoid muscles, and may cause difficulty in walking up steps, getting up from a chair, and combing the hair. A rapid, coarse hand tremor is also characteristic. The many subjective and objective findings are also congruent with old age, making it imperative that the diagnosis be based on a series of thyroid function studies before therapy is initiated.

Management

Treatment in hyperthyroidism is based on decreasing the hormone production of the gland, which can be achieved by surgically removing a portion of the gland, administering radioactive iodine to destroy a portion of the gland, or using a medication that will suppress the functioning of the gland.

The treatment of choice in older persons is radioactive iodine, which can lead to the development of hypothyroidism. The antithyroid drugs methimazole and propylthiouracil may be used to produce a euthyroid state, but the incidence of major side effects and the length of time the medications must be taken may not make them the treatment of choice. Producing a euthyroid state with a course of antithyroid drug therapy followed by radio-active iodine is recommended (Davis, 1977). Because radioactive iodine does not reach its peak effect for several months, supplemental antithyroid therapy may be needed during this period.

Antithyroid drugs
Methimazole and propylthiouracil

Drug action. Methimazole and propylthiouracil block biosynthesis of thyroid function, probably by inhibiting the oxidative enzymes that catalyze the iodination and coupling processes in the formation of thyroxine and liothyronine.

Drug	Dosage
Methimazole	Initial (based on extent of hyperthyroidism): 15 to 60 mg daily in three doses at 8-hour intervals. Maintenance: 5 to 30 mg in two to three divided doses.
Propylthiouracil	Initial: 300 to 1200 mg in three divided doses at 8-hour intervals or four divided doses at 6-hour intervals. Maintenance: 50 to 800 mg in two to four divided doses.

Proper use and precautions
1. The medication must be taken exactly as directed and not discontinued without consultation with the physician.
2. The medication must be taken every day in regularly spaced doses (around the clock).
3. The medication is to be taken at the same time daily in relation to meals, because foods can alter the response to the medication.
4. In case of surgery, injury, infection, or illness of any kind, the physician should be notified because of the risk of thyrotoxicosis.
5. When the medication is given before radioactive iodine therapy, it should be discontinued 3 to 4 days before administration of radioactive iodine. This action will prevent impairment of radioactive iodine uptake. The treatment may be resumed 3 to 5 days later until a euthyroid state is achieved.
6. Drug interactions that may occur include oral anticoagulants and heparin (increase anticoagulant effect) and agranulocytosis-producing medications (increase the risk of this disorder).
7. Side effects that require immediate attention include fever, chills, sore throat, yellowing of eyes and skin, loss of hearing, enlarged lymph

nodes, unusual bleeding or bruising, increase or decrease in urination, backache, edema of lower extremities, and symptoms of hypothyroidism or hyperthyroidism. Other side effects that may occur include itching; dizziness; joint pain; loss of taste; nausea and vomiting; numbness or tingling of fingers, toes, or face; skin rash; darkening of skin; or loss or lightening of hair.

8. Monitoring includes regular physician visits, thyroid function studies, liver function tests, total and differential leukocyte counts, and observation for signs and symptoms of overdosage or underdosage.

REFERENCES

Andres, R., and others: Diabetes and aging, Hosp. Pract. **2:**63, 1967.

Davis, P.J.: Endocrines and aging, Hosp. Pract. **12:**113, 1977.

Eliopoulous, C.: Diagnosis and management of diabetes in the elderly, Am. J. Nurs. **78:**884, 1978.

Guthrie, D.W., and Guthrie, R.A.: Nursing management of diabetes mellitus, ed. 2, St. Louis, 1982, The C.V. Mosby Co.

Hayter, J.: Diabetes and aging, Geriatr. Nurs. **2**(1):32, 1981.

Larner, J.: Insulin and oral hypoglycemic agents. In Goodman, L.S., and others, editors: The pharmacological basis of therapeutics, ed. 6, New York, 1980, Macmillan Publishing Co., Inc.

Lundin, D.: Reporting urine test results switching from + to %, Am. J. Nurs. **78:**878, 1978.

National Diabetes Information Clearing House: Diabetes and aging, Pub. No. 81-2178, Washington, D.C., 1980, National Institutes of Health.

SUGGESTED READINGS

Shagan, B.: Is diabetes a model for aging? Med. Clin. North Am. **60:**1209, 1976.

Skillman, T., and Falko, J.: Recognizing thyroid disease in the elderly: current considerations, Geriatrics **36:**63, 1981.

Todd, B.: Drugs and the elderly: when the patient is taking a sulfonylurea, Geriatr. Nurs. **2**(4):149, 1981.

Turnbridge, W.: Is hypothyroidism causing your patient's lethargy? Geriatrics **36:**79, 1981.

11

MANAGEMENT OF SELECTED CARDIOVASCULAR PROBLEMS

The stress placed on the cardiovascular system throughout life makes it very vulnerable to pathological changes as persons grow older. These changes, which are frequently referred to as diseases of life-style, are primarily preventable if a program of prevention is practiced throughout life. A well-balanced diet, physical fitness, and stress management promote healthy cardiac functioning. Problems that are discussed in this chapter include coronary heart disease, congestive heart failure, arrhythmia, hypertension, and peripheral vascular disease. Management is limited to drug therapy.

CORONARY HEART DISEASE

Coronary heart disease is the most important cardiovascular disease of the older adult and one of the most serious in contemporary society. The Framingham Heart Study (Kannel, 1976) shows a marked increase of coronary artery disease and myocardial infarction with advancing age.

In persons with coronary heart disease, the coronary arterial channels become too narrow to transport the amount of blood needed to meet the demands of the myocardium for oxygen under a variety of circumstances. The underlying reason for the narrowing of the coronary arteries is atherosclerosis. The atherosclerotic process remains asymptomatic for several decades, but beginning at about the fifth to sixth decade, symptoms begin to occur. In this process, lipids are laid down on the intima, which is the inner lining of the coronary vessels. These fatty deposits on the blood vessel wall interfere with the blood flow to the myocardium. The blood vessels, which begin to harden, lose their ability to dilate adequately in response to the need for more oxygenated blood required during physical activity.

Atherosclerosis is a multifactorial disease. Factors playing a role in the development of the lesions include a diet high in saturated fats and cholesterol, emotional stress, physical inactivity, hypertension, diabetes, smoking, hyperlipidemia, and heredity. Alterations in life-style that will decrease these etiological factors should have a positive effect on the cardiovascular status of future generations as they grow older.

Signs and symptoms

The major clinical manifestation of the myocardial ischemia and hypoxia that occur in persons with coronary heart disease associated with atherosclerosis is chest pain or pressure sensation. The pain, which is caused by a lack of sufficient oxygenated blood to the myocardium, varies in severity and duration and generally begins under the sternum, radiating to the throat. It may be referred to the jaw, back of the neck, and both arms. However, the older person is more likely to have atypical features. A frequent difference is the substitution of dyspnea on exertion for chest pain. The dyspnea that is associated with a feeling of tightness of the chest does not produce orthopnea or paroxysmal nocturnal dyspnea. Other patients may have atypical pain that resembles other health problems. Paroxysmal epigastric pain may resemble the discomfort of an ulcer or hiatal hernia. In other patients angina may manifest itself as recurrent left shoulder or wrist pain or a tightness of the neck that can be mistaken for arthritis. Because of changes in pain perception, the pain may not follow a prescribed pattern or may not be perceived. Patients reporting the typical or atypical pain should be referred to a physician for diagnosis.

Management

Management of angina pectoris involves weight control, a diet low in saturated fats, a balance of rest and activity, cessation of smoking, stress management, and avoidance of precipitating circumstances. Drug management of coronary artery disease focuses on the use of vasodilators, β-adrenergic blockers, and calcium channel inhibitors to prevent or relieve the pain associated with angina pectoris. The use of drugs to lower cholesterol and triglyceride levels, which are frequently elevated in persons with coronary artery disease, is not recommended for older patients because of serious side effects and has not been proved to decrease mortality and morbidity from coronary artery disease.

Coronary vasodilators

Drug action. Antianginal agents, or coronary vasodilators, used to treat the problems of coronary heart disease in older adults produce their effect by two major actions: (1) improving the blood flow through the coronary vessels, thereby relieving the ischemia and hypoxia, and (2) decreasing the work load of the heart, which reduces the need for oxygen.

Drug	Dosage
Nitroglycerin	
Oral	
Extended-release capsules	2.5 to 9.0 mg q.12h.; may be increased to q.8h.
Extended-release tablets	1.3 to 6.5 mg q.12h.; may be increased to q.8h.
Sublingual	
Tablets	0.15 to 0.6 mg repeated at 5 minute intervals. If relief is not obtained after a total of three tablets, physician should be contacted or patient taken to a hospital.
Topical	
Ointment, 2%	2.5 to 5 cm q.3-4h. during daytime and at bedtime.
Transdermal infusion system	2.5 to 10 mg q.24h. One 10 cm^2 surface area system delivers 5 mg of nitroglycerin over 24 hours.

Proper use and precautions

1. Medication should be stored in a cool, dry place (not in the refrigerator) in original tightly closed container.
2. Alcoholic beverages must be avoided, because they may cause serious hypotension.
3. The medication should not be suddenly discontinued if it has been taken for several weeks. This action may cause sudden attacks of angina.
4. Side effects that may occur include skin rash, dizziness, fainting (orthostatic hypotension), flushing of face and neck, headache, nausea, vomiting, and visual disturbances. Side effects may diminish as the body becomes accustomed to the medication.
5. Drug interactions that may occur include alcohol, antihypertensives, vasodilators (may intensify orthostatic effects of nitroglycerin), or sympathomimetics (may reduce antianginal effects).
6. Tolerance may occur after prolonged use.
7. Monitoring includes blood pressure, heart rate, cardiac function, and headache frequency.
8. Implications for specific drugs:
   a. Nitroglycerin extended-release capsules and tablets.
      (1) Medication is used to prevent attacks.

    (2) Absorption is variable.

    (3) Medication should be taken with a full glass of water on an empty stomach (1 hour before meals or 2 hours after meals).

  b. Nitroglycerin sublingual tablets.

    (1) Medication is used to relieve pain during an attack.

    (2) Patient should sit down when taking medication. If dizziness occurs, the patient should be instructed to take a few deep breaths or bend forward.

    (3) Medication acts in 1 to 5 minutes and can be repeated as directed by physician.

    (4) Because deterioration of this medication can occur, its strength should be tested every 3 to 4 weeks by placing a tablet under the tongue. Burning or tingling of the tongue and flushing of the face will occur if the tablets are effective.

    (5) Medication should always be stored in original glass bottle.

  c. Nitroglycerin ointment.

    (1) Medication is used to prevent attacks.

    (2) Instructions must be carefully followed, using dose preparation papers that are then used to apply the ointment to the skin. The ointment is spread in a thin, even layer without rubbing or massaging.

    (3) Site of application is the nonhairy skin of the chest, stomach, front of the thighs, or other accessible skin.

    (4) Sites of application should be rotated.

  d. Nitroglycerin transdermal system.

    (1) Medication is not intended for immediate relief of attacks.

    (2) Instructions must be carefully followed. The adhesive surface of the system is applied to the selected skin site as with the ointment application.

    (3) Contact with water will not affect the system.

Drug	Dosage
Isosorbide dinitrate	
Tablets	5 to 10 mg q.6h.
Chewable tablets	5 to 10 mg q.2-3h.
Extended-release tablets or capsules	40 mg q.12h. with increases up to 40 mg q.6h.
Sublingual tablets	5 to 10 mg q.2-3h.

Proper use and precautions

1. Medication should be stored in a cool dry place (not in the refrigerator) in a tightly closed container.

2. Alcoholic beverages should be avoided, because they may cause severe hypotension.
3. Medication should not be suddenly discontinued if it has been taken for several weeks.
4. Tolerance may occur after prolonged use. Patients should be advised that this development is not to be confused with addiction.
5. Side effects that may occur include skin rash, dizziness, fainting (orthostatic hypotension), flushing of face and neck, prolonged or serious headaches, and nausea or vomiting. Side effects may diminish as body becomes accustomed to medication.
6. Light-headedness that may occur when the patient is coming to an upright position can be relieved by moving slowly and remaining in a sitting position for a brief period.
7. Drug interactions that may occur include alcohol, antihypertensives, vasodilators (may intensify orthostatic hypotension), and sympathomimetics (may reduce antianginal effects.)
8. Monitoring includes blood pressure, cardiac function, and frequency of headaches.
9. Implications for specific drugs:
   a. Extended-release capsules or tablets.
      (1) Medication is used to prevent attacks.
      (2) Medication should be taken with a full glass of water on an empty stomach (1 hour before or 2 hours after meals).
      (3) Medication should not be broken or chewed.
   b. Chewable or sublingual tablets.
      (1) Medication is used to relieve acute attacks while patient is taking other oral dosage forms. It may be used before anticipated stress to prevent an attack.
      (2) Patient should sit down and take medicine as directed (chewable or sublingual). If pain is not relieved by three tablets after 30 minutes, immediate medical care must be sought.
      (3) Chewable form must be chewed well and held in the mouth at least 2 minutes.
      (4) Relief with sublingual form should be achieved in 2 to 5 minutes. Action of the chewable form is 5 to 10 minutes.

β-Adrenergic blocker
Propranolol

Drug action. Propranolol is a β-adrenergic receptor blocking drug. Blocking β-adrenergic receptor sites with drugs produces a decrease in heart rate, cardiac output, and blood pressure; also see section on Hypertension. Propranolol is indicated in patients with moderate to severe angina pectoris who have not responded to preventive measures and nitrate therapy.

Drug	Dosage
Propranolol	Initially 10 to 20 mg three to four times a day. Increase dosage at 3 to 7 day intervals until optimum response is obtained.

Proper use and precautions
1. See Hypertension.
2. Because of the potential for adverse effects, therapy should be evaluated frequently.

Calcium channel inhibitors
Nifedipine

Drug action. Nifedipine is an antianginal drug belonging to a new class of compounds known as calcium channel inhibitors. The contractile ability of the cardiac and vascular smooth muscle depends on the movement of extracellular calcium ions into the muscle cells through specific ion channels. Nifedipine, by selectively inhibiting the influx of calcium ions across the cell membrane of cardiac and vascular smooth muscle, produces vascular relaxation, inhibition of coronary artery spasm, and reduction of oxygen use.

Drug	Dosage
Nifedipine capsules	10 mg three times a day. May be increased if necessary, but more than 120 mg/day rarely needed.

Proper use and precautions
1. Sublingual nitroglycerin may be used to control acute angina during nifedipine titration.
2. Excessive hypotension may be a problem that is sometimes related to dosage. Light-headedness that may occur when the person is coming to an upright position can be relieved by moving slowly and remaining in a sitting position for a brief period.
3. β-Adrenergic blockers such as propranolol should not be withdrawn abruptly, but dosage should be reduced gradually before nifedipine therapy is begun. Concurrent therapy with β-adrenergic blockers may be beneficial if blood pressure is carefully monitored.
4. Drug may increase digoxin levels, requiring careful monitoring and digoxin dosage alteration.
5. Side effects that may occur include dizziness, flushing, peripheral edema, heat sensation, headache, and nausea.
6. Monitoring includes regular physician visits, blood pressure, and cardiac function.

Verapamil

Drug action. Verapamil is an inhibitor of calcium ion influx, producing relaxation, preventing coronary artery spasm, and reducing oxygen use.

Drug	Dosage
Verapamil tablets	Initial: 80 mg three to four times a day. May be increased at daily or weekly intervals if necessary but more than 320 to 480 mg/day rarely needed.

Proper use and precautions
1. See Nifedipine.
2. Verapamil is contraindicated in severe left-sided ventricular failure, hypotension (systolic pressure less than 90 mm Hg), sick sinus syndrome, and second- or third-degree atrioventricular block.
3. During the first week of therapy, verapamil increases digoxin levels by 50% to 70%, which can cause digitalis toxicity. The daily dose of digoxin should be reduced and the patient carefully monitored.

CONGESTIVE HEART FAILURE

Heart failure is defined as an inability of the heart to pump blood at a rate adequate to meet tissue metabolic demands. Inefficient pump action may be caused by damage to the heart muscle as a result of ischemia, infarction, hypertension, or arrhythmias.

Signs and symptoms

Older patients may not have the classic manifestations of congestive heart failure that are exhibited by younger persons. Early symptoms that are often not recognized include weakness, fatigue, mental confusion, forgetfulness, and mild pulmonary symptoms. Classic symptoms that may be present include dyspnea, orthopnea, paroxysmal nocturnal dyspnea, coughing, hemoptysis, and wheezing. Insomnia may be reported by the patient, but when sleeping behavior is described by the family, it resembles Cheyne-Stokes respirations. Gastrointestinal symptoms that may be present include lack of appetite, nausea and vomiting, and abdominal discomfort. Edema occurs as the disease progresses.

Management

The mainstays of treatment are the cardiac glycosides, of which digoxin is the most commonly prescribed, and diuretics (see drug description under

Hypertension). Vasodilators, with or without digoxin, are also used to treat congestive heart failure. Treatment does not differ from that of younger patients, but older patients are particularly susceptible to drug problems.

In general, dosage of cardiac glycosides should be lower for elderly patients than for younger ones. Creatinine clearance, which is greatly reduced in older patients, correlates with digoxin clearance and is used in dose adjustment. Decreased body size, reduced renal function, electrolyte imbalance, and vascular disease contribute to the very narrow difference between the therapeutic and toxic digoxin dose in the elderly. Symptoms of digoxin toxicity may be different in elderly than in younger patients. Frequently, psychiatric disturbances such as confusion ("digoxin delirium") and depression occur. Common warning signs of nausea, vomiting, and bradycardia are often absent. Changes in cardiac rhythm and a worsening of the heart failure may be manifestations of digoxin overdose.

The need for digoxin therapy must be carefully assessed and the dose individually titrated and monitored. Often a diuretic alone will be adequate to treat congestive heart failure in many older patients. A discussion of diuretics is included under Hypertension.

Cardiac glycosides

Drug action. The two main types of pharmacological actions on the heart are (1) increased strength of the heartbeat and (2) altered electrophysiological properties of the heart, thereby affecting the rate and the rhythm.

Drug	Dosage
Digoxin (oral)	Maintenance: 0.125 mg to 0.5 mg daily (geriatric patients may require smaller dosages because of impaired renal function and small stature).

Proper use and precautions
1. Medication should be taken exactly as prescribed at the same time every day.
2. Pulse should be taken regularly, and a health professional should be contacted if rate becomes slower or rhythm irregular.
3. Medication should not be discontinued without consulting the physician.
4. Before the patient has any surgery, the doctor or dentist should be informed about this medication.
5. Prescribed and over-the-counter medications should not be taken without consultation with the physician.
6. Drug interactions may occur with a wide variety of drugs. Consult Chapter 4.

7. Side effects that may occur include slow or irregular pulse, loss of appetite, nausea or vomiting, weakness (report immediately), blurred vision, changes in color perception, diarrhea, and confusion. Cardiotoxicity may develop in the absence of gastrointestinal symptoms.

8. Monitoring includes regular physician visits, pulse, blood pressure, cardiac function, vision tests for color perception changes, hepatic and renal function, serum electrolytes, and digoxin serum concentration.

ARRHYTHMIA

The incidence of arrhythmias and conduction disturbances increases with age. These problems are frequently caused by angina, coronary insufficiency, hypokalemia related to diuretic therapy, and digitalis therapy. The risk is also high for adults when barium enemas and other diagnostic studies require enema preparation that may cause dehydration. Heart block caused by fibrosis in the conducting system is common in the elderly and manifested by a decrease in effort tolerance and Stokes-Adams attacks.

Signs and symptoms

Because arrhythmias may be caused by various cardiac pathological changes, may be present with or without symptoms, and are diagnosed by skilled practitioners, this discussion will be limited to symptoms that may be reported to the practitioner by the patient or family. Symptoms that may be reported include palpitations, irregular heartbeat, very slow to rapid heart rate, apprehension, dizziness, and loss of consciousness. Sophisticated technology is used in the diagnosis of these abnormalities.

Management

Many patients do not require therapy. When treatment is necessary, the use of a cardiac pacemaker is usually most successful. Atrial fibrillation is also common in older adults and responds to digitalization. Ventricular arrhythmias associated with myocardial infarction are most commonly treated with antiarrhythmic drugs such as quinidine, procainamide, and disopyramide.

Disopyramide may cause or complicate congestive heart failure or produce severe hypotension because of negative inotropic properties. Because it has anticholinergic properties, the drug may cause urinary retention and is used with caution for patients susceptible to glaucoma. Propranolol also has antiarrhythmic action but is often avoided for the elderly, because even small doses may cause marked bradycardia and hypotension.

Antiarrhythmics are difficult drugs to use because of frequent side effects, the need for precise dosing intervals, and poor correlation between serum level data and drug action. The value of treatment must be carefully weighed against the risk of therapy.

Antiarrhythmics

Quinidine and procainamide, the drugs of choice in the treatment of certain kinds of arrhythmias and considered reliable forms of treatment for ambulatory patients, will be discussed in this section.

Quinidine

Drug action. The action of quinidine includes reduction of excitability of the myocardium, depression of pacemaker activity, and prolongation of the refractory period of cardiac repolarization. As a result of these actions, beats of ventricular and atrioventricular origin and ventricular tachycardia are corrected.

Drug	Dosage
Quinidine sulfate capsules and tablets	100 to 300 mg three to six times daily.
Quinidine sulfate extended-release tablets	300 to 600 mg q.8-12h.
Quinidine gluconate extended-release tablets	324 to 648 mg q.6-12h.

Proper use and precautions
1. Dosages may need to be decreased because of accumulation of metabolites in persons with decreased renal function.
2. The medication should not be discontinued without consultation with the physician or other health professional.
3. Medication is to be taken with a full glass of water on an empty stomach (1 hour before or 2 hours after meals). If medication causes gastric upset, it may be taken with milk or food.
4. Before the patient has any type of surgery, the physician or dentist should be notified regarding this medication.
5. Drug interactions that may occur include antiarrhythmics, anticoagulants, barbiturates, phenytoin (may decrease quinidine serum levels), cholinergics (may decrease cholinergic effects), digoxin and other cardiac glycosides (may increase serum digoxin levels), neuromuscular blocking agents (blocking effects may be increased or prolonged), potassium-containing medication (may increase effect of quinidine), and urinary alkalizers (increases potential for toxic effects).
6. Side effects that may occur include visual changes, dizziness, tinnitus,

severe headache, fainting (orthostatic hypotension), fever, rash, itching, breathing problems, rapid pulse, unusual bleeding or bruising,
bitter taste, loss of appetite, nausea, diarrhea, stomach pain, and mental confusion.

7. If any side effects are noted after the first few doses, the physician
   should be contacted immediately, since hypersensitivity to the drug
   may occur.
8. Carrying an identification card indicating that this medication is being
   taken is recommended.
9. Monitoring includes cardiac function, serum quinidine concentration
   determinations (with doses over 2 gm daily), blood cell counts, and
   hepatic and renal function tests.

Procainamide

Drug action. Procainamide acts similarly to quinidine by suppressing
automaticity in ectopic tissues and by slowing conduction in atrial and ventricular musculature and in the specialized transmission system; it is used as
an antiarrhythmic for patients who cannot tolerate quinidine. Therapy is
often limited by adverse effects.

Drug	Dosage
Procainamide capsules Procainamide tablets	Atrial antiarrhythmic maintenance: 500 mg to 1 gm four to six times a day.
	Ventricular antiarrhythmic maintenance: 250 to 500 mg q.3h.
	Antimyotonic: 250 mg two times a day.

Proper use and precautions
1. Medication should be stored in a tightly closed container in a dry place
   (not in the refrigerator).
2. Drug should be taken with a glass of water on an empty stomach (1
   hour before or 2 hours after meals).
3. If medication causes gastric upset, it can be taken with milk or food.
4. Drug interactions that may occur include antihypertensives (may increase hypotensive effects), cholinergics (may inhibit effect on striated
   muscles), neuromuscular blocking agents (blocking effects may be increased or prolonged), and other antiarrhythmics (may produce additive effects).
5. Before the patient has any surgery or emergency treatment, the physician should be notified regarding this medication.
6. Side effects that may occur include fever, itching, joint pain, painful
   breathing, skin rash (typical of lupus erythematosus), fatigue, sore

throat, unusual bleeding or bruising, hallucinations, and mental confusion or depression.

7. Monitoring includes blood pressure, cardiac function, blood cell counts, and complaints of joint pains and malaise suggestive of systemic lupus erythematosus.

HYPERTENSION

Hypertension means excessive pressure. It may refer to increased pressure in any blood vessel but usually refers to elevated mean systemic arterial or diastolic blood pressure. Diastolic hypertension occurs as a result of arteriolar constriction. A diastolic pressure greater than 90 mm Hg is defined as hypertension, because at this value renal function is endangered, and the frequency of complications tends to rise significantly. Systolic hypertension may also occur as a result of increased rigidity of the large arterial vessels. When systolic hypertension is treated, pressure should be reduced gradually over several weeks to prevent sudden blood pressure reduction, which could significantly reduce cerebral blood flow and lead to cerebrovascular thrombosis.

Hypertension is a major risk factor for atherosclerosis and cardiovascular complications such as congestive heart failure, myocardial infarction, and angina pectoris. Sustained hypertension results in organ damage to the eyes, brain, heart, and kidneys. Hypertension is slightly more common in males than in females and twice as common in blacks as whites. Mortality increases with age.

Unless organ damage is already present, the diagnosis of hypertension should be based on the documentation of several determinations of blood pressure before drug therapy is started.

Signs and symptoms

Hypertension, frequently referred to as the "silent disease," has no characteristic signs and symptoms. Most patients feel well, and the abnormal blood pressure may be identified when the person is seeking other health care. Headaches, commonly reported as a symptom of high blood pressure, are not consistently present. Symptoms generally do not occur until organ or vessel damage occurs.

Management

Recent studies have suggested that the treatment of even mild degrees of hypertension is effective in lowering mortality from cardiovascular disease.

The treatment of hypertension in the older adult continues to be controversial even though the risks are recognized. The benefits of treatment must be weighed carefully against the side effects of the drugs used and the possibility of reduced cardiac output and cerebral insufficiency producing greater hazards. The likelihood of good compliance is poor unless the benefits of adhering to the treatment plan are carefully explained and monitored. As few different medications and as few doses per day as possible will be helpful in preventing therapeutic failure.

Other treatment methods should be tried before drug therapy. Reduced salt intake, weight reduction, relaxation therapy, and regular exercise have been effective in lowering blood pressure in mild hypertension. Once drug therapy has been determined to be necessary, the stepped-care approach is used, in which an easy-to-use, relatively inexpensive drug, such as a diuretic, is chosen. If it is not effective, another drug (step 2) is added, with additive effects. Sometimes a third step is needed.

Diuretics
Thiazides

Drug action. Thiazides increase renal excretion of sodium and chloride and an accompanying volume of water. A significant excretion of potassium also occurs.

Drug	Dosage
Hydrochlorothiazide	25 to 100 mg in one or two doses a day.
Benzthiazide	50 to 200 mg in two to four doses a day.
Polythiazide	2 to 4 mg in one daily dose.
Chlorthalidone	25 to 100 mg in one daily dose.
Numerous others	

Proper use and precautions
1. Medicine should be taken at the same time each day. The last dose should be taken no later than 6 PM to keep the increase in urine from affecting nighttime sleep.
2. Unusual fatigue may be observed early in the course of treatment.
3. Drug may cause loss of potassium and require foods rich in potassium or a potassium supplement. Signs of potassium loss include thirst, dry mouth, irregular heartbeat, weak pulse, mental changes, muscle cramps, nausea, vomiting, and unusual weakness or fatigue.
4. Other side effects include hyperglycemia, hyperuricemia, increased sensitivity to sunlight, skin rash or hives, sore throat or fever, unusual bleeding or bruising, yellowing of eyes or skin, orthostatic hypotension, and loss of appetite.
5. Patients allergic to sulfonamide-type medications may be allergic to thiazides.

6. Drug interactions that may occur include anticoagulants (effects decreased), antigout drugs (raise uric acid levels), other antihypertensive agents or skeletal muscle relaxants (their effects may be potentiated), cardiac glycosides (may increase potential for digitalis toxicity), hypoglycemics (thiazide may raise blood glucose levels), lithium (increases potential for lithium toxicity), and methenamine (its effectiveness decreases).
7. Monitoring includes serum electrolyte determination, daily weight, and blood pressure.

Furosemide

Drug action. Furosemide inhibits active chloride transport over the entire length of the ascending loop of Henle (a loop diuretic).

Drug	Dosage
Furosemide	20 to 80 mg daily.

Proper use and precautions
1. Furosemide is the drug of choice in hypertension associated with renal insufficiency.
2. Adverse effects are similar to those of the thiazides.
3. Monitoring includes blood pressure, serum electrolyte determination, and daily weight.

Potassium-sparing diuretics
Spironolactone

Drug action. Spironolactone is an aldosterone antagonist.

Drug	Dosage
Spironolactone	25 mg two to four times a day.

Proper use and precautions
1. Medication may cause hyperkalemia, especially for patients with impaired renal function.
2. Onset of action is gradual, and 4 to 5 days are required to achieve the full diuretic effect.
3. Spironolactone is most frequently used in combination with a thiazide (e.g., Aldactazide).
4. Medication is contraindicated for patients receiving digoxin, because concurrent use elevates digoxin plasma levels and may induce digoxin toxicity.
5. Other side effects include drowsiness, skin rash, mental confusion, and gynecomastia.

6. Monitoring includes blood pressure, serum electrolyte determination, and daily weight.

Triamterene

Drug action. Triamterene inhibits reabsorption of sodium and chloride.

Drug	Dosage
Triamterene	100 mg every other day to 300 mg daily.

Proper use and precautions
1. Triamterene conserves potassium and therefore should not be used with potassium supplements.
2. Triamterene is often used in combination with a thiazide (e.g., Dyazide).
3. The usual dose should be taken after meals.
4. Monitoring includes blood pressure, serum electrolyte determination, and daily weight.

Amiloride

Drug action. Amiloride conserves potassium.

Drug	Dosage
Amiloride	5 mg daily to a maximum of 10 mg daily.

Proper use and precautions
1. Amiloride is most often used in combination with a thiazide (e.g., Moduretic).
2. Medication may cause hyperkalemia, especially in the elderly.
3. Medication should be administered with food.
4. Monitoring includes blood pressure, serum electrolyte determination, and daily weight.

Peripheral adrenergic blocking agents
Propranolol

Drug action. Propranolol is a β-adrenergic blocking agent that produces slow but balanced reductions in elevated systolic and diastolic pressures.

Drug	Dosage
Propranolol	First day: 40 to 160 mg in 2 to 4 hours. Maintenance: 120 to 480 mg in two doses.

Proper use and precautions
1. Drug should be taken with meals or immediately following meals.
2. Pulse is taken regularly. A slower than usual rate may indicate a circulation problem.

3. Caution is necessary when driving or doing work requiring alertness because of drowsiness.
4. Drug is relatively contraindicated for patients with bronchial asthma, hay fever, congestive heart failure, and bradycardia; also contraindicated is the concurrent use of tricyclic antidepressants and oral hypoglycemic agents.
5. Sudden withdrawal can be dangerous, because it can cause increased angina, arrhythmias, myocardial infarction, and even death.
6. Before the patient has any surgery or emergency medical treatment, the doctor or dentist should be informed about this medication.
7. Carrying an identification card indicating that the medication is being taken is recommended.
8. Pharmacokinetic and pharmacological properties cause numerous interaction possibilities. See Chapter 4.
9. Side effects include fatigue, bradycardia, hallucinations, dizziness, reduced alertness, hypoglycemia, bronchospasm, acute pulmonary edema, and gastrointestinal upset.
10. Monitoring includes blood pressure; pulse rate; blood cell counts; blood glucose (for diabetic patients); and cardiac, liver, and kidney functions.

Metoprolol

Drug action. Metoprolol is similar to propranolol. In low doses it causes less blockade of the β_2 receptors of the bronchi and blood vessels.

Drug	Dosage
Metoprolol	Initial: 100 mg in two doses.
	Maintenance: 100 to 450 mg in two doses.

Proper use and precautions. See Propranolol.

Nadolol

Drug action. Nadolol is similar to propranolol. It is excreted unchanged in the urine and has a half-life of 14 to 20 hours in patients with normal renal function. Only one dose daily is required.

Drug	Dosage
Nadolol	Initial: 40 mg in one dose.
	Maintenance: 80 to 320 mg in one dose.

Proper use and precautions
1. See Propranolol.
2. Dosage reduction may be required for older adults with impaired renal function.

Reserpine

Drug action. Reserpine produces a partial depletion of norepinephrine in the sympathetic postganglionic nerves.

Drug	Dosage
Reserpine	0.1 to 0.25 mg in one dose.

Proper use and precautions
1. Effects of the drug are not fully manifested for several days to 2 weeks and may persist for as long as 4 weeks after discontinuation.
2. Drug is often used concurrently with a thiazide or hydralazine.
3. Drug should be used with caution for patients with decreased alertness and is contraindicated for persons with a history of mental depression or ulcerative colitis.
4. Side effects are numerous and include drowsiness, nasal stuffiness, gastrointestinal disturbances, nightmares, and psychic depression.
5. Monitoring includes blood pressure, cardiac function, and mood changes.

Guanethidine

Drug action. Guanethidine depletes adrenergic nerves of norepinephrine and prevents release of that which remains; this action results in vasodilatation and a decrease in plasma renin activity.

Drug	Dosage
Guanethidine	10 to 300 mg in one dose.

Proper use and precautions
1. Onset of action is a few hours to a few days for full effect, and duration of action may be 4 or more days. Dosage increases should not be made more often than every 5 to 7 days.
2. Guanethidine is reserved for use in hypertension resistant to other drugs because of the frequency and severity of adverse effects.
3. Side effects include orthostatic hypotension, edema, diarrhea, and breathing difficulty.
4. Patient should be cautioned to move slowly when coming from a recumbent to upright position.
5. Caution must be used during hot weather and in consuming alcohol, exercising, and standing long periods, all of which contribute to vasodilatation.
6. Drug interactions are common and include CNS depressants, phenothiazines, tricyclic antidepressants, and hypoglycemic medications.
7. Drug should be withdrawn 2 weeks before surgery. If emergency sur-

gery is required, anesthetics and preanesthetic agents should be administered with caution.

8. Combination therapy with thiazides and hydralazine is indicated in some patients and requires individual titration to determine the lowest possible therapeutic dose of each drug.

9. Monitoring includes blood pressure, cardiac function, and renal function.

Prazosin

Drug action. Prazosin blocks α-adrenergic receptors, and this blocking results in vasodilatation.

Drug	Dosage
Prazosin	First day: 1 mg at bedtime. Maintenance: 1 to 20 mg in two doses.

Proper use and precautions

1. Treatment must begin slowly and dosage adjustments made gradually to avoid severe postural hypotension with syncope.

2. Hypotensive syncope can be avoided if the first dose is small (1 mg or less) and given at bedtime with instructions to the patient not to get up for 3 hours.

3. Side effects include palpitations, dizziness, nasal stuffiness, edema, drowsiness, and anticholinergic effects.

4. The dose should be decreased to 1 or 2 mg three times a day when a diuretic or another antihypertensive drug is added and further upward adjustments made gradually if needed.

5. Monitoring includes blood pressure, heart rate, serum electrolyte determination, and renal function.

Methyldopa

Drug action. Methyldopa is enzymatically converted to a false transmitter (α-methylnorepinephrine), which displaces the natural transmitter in adrenergic nerve endings. Effective transmission of nerve impulses is blocked, and there is a resulting decrease in blood pressure because of a reduction in sympathetic tone.

Drug	Dosage
Methyldopa	Initial: 250 mg two to three times a day for 2 days. Maintenance: 500 mg to 2 gm a day divided into two to four doses.

Proper use and precautions

1. Drowsiness is a common side effect. Tolerance to the sedative effects

often develops within a few weeks. Upward dosage adjustments should be initiated with the bedtime dose to minimize the sedative effects.

2. Caution is recommended when getting up suddenly from a lying or sitting position.
3. Methyldopa therapy may produce a positive direct antiglobulin (Coombs') test; liver disorders characterized by fever, malaise, and occasional jaundice; and hemolytic anemia. Baseline laboratory studies should be done before therapy is started.
4. Monitoring includes blood pressure, serum electrolyte determinations, temperature, weight, cardiac function, renal function, liver function, and blood cell count.

Clonidine

Drug action. Clonidine stimulates α-adrenergic receptors, and this stimulation results in a decrease in sympathetic activity by inhibiting vasoconstrictor centers.

Drug	Dosage
Clonidine	Initial: 0.1 mg two times a day. Maintenance: 0.1 or 0.2 mg two to four times daily.

Proper use and precautions
1. Drowsiness and dry mouth are common side effects.
2. The drug should not be discontinued abruptly, and patients should be cautioned not to discontinue therapy without medical supervision because of the possibility of severe rebound hypertension. A second prescription should be carried for emergency use to ensure continuous therapy.
3. Combination therapy with diuretics or other antihypertensive agents is indicated in some patients and requires individual titration to determine the lowest possible therapeutic dose of each drug.
4. Interactions occur with alcohol and other CNS depressants (increase depression), other antihypertensives, diuretics (increase antihypertensive effects), propranolol (discontinuance following concurrent use may increase risk of clonidine withdrawal hypertensive crisis), and tricyclic antidepressants (decrease hypotensive effects).
5. Monitoring consists of blood pressure and ophthalmoscopic examinations in long-term therapy.

Arteriolar dilators
Hydralazine

Drug action. Hydralazine causes vasodilatation through an unknown mechanism of action.

Drug	Dosage
Hydralazine	Initial: 10 mg four times a day for the first 2 to 4 days; 25 mg four times a day for the balance of the week and 50 mg four times a day for the second and subsequent weeks.
	Maintenance: adjustment to lowest effective level.

Proper use and precautions

1. Combination with β-adrenergic blocking agents such as propranolol will minimize some side effects such as tachycardia, headache, and dizziness.
2. Systemic lupus erythematosus–like syndrome occurs more frequently in patients receiving greater than 200 mg/day, in slow acetylators (acetylation is the major route of hydralazine metabolism), and in patients with impaired renal function.
3. Medication should be withdrawn gradually to avoid a sudden increase in blood pressure.
4. Monitoring includes blood pressure, cardiac function, renal function, and blood cell counts.

Minoxidil

Drug action. Minoxidil causes vasodilatation through an unknown mechanism of action.

Drug	Dosage
Minoxidil	Initial: 5 mg first day.
	Maintenance: 20 to 40 mg a day; maximum recommended daily dosage is 100 mg.

Proper use and precautions

1. Minoxidil is used for patients in whom hypertension cannot be controlled by other drugs.
2. Drug produces reflex tachycardia and palpitations, which can be suppressed by the coadministration of a β-blocker.
3. Drug causes salt and water retention, requiring adequate diuretic therapy, usually with furosemide.
4. Drug causes hair growth (hypertrichosis) on face and body, which is usually reversible.

Angiotensin-converting enzyme inhibitors
Captopril

Drug action. Captopril, by competitively inhibiting angiotensin-converting enzyme and thereby the conversion of angiotensin I to angiotensin II, causes lowering of blood pressure.

Drug	Dosage
Captopril	Initial: 25 mg t.i.d. Adjustments may be made every 1 to 2 weeks until satisfactory. Range: 25 to 150 mg t.i.d.

Proper use and precautions
1. Drug should be administered 1 hour before meals.
2. It is indicated for treatment of hypertensive patients who have failed to respond satisfactorily to other drugs or who have developed unacceptable side effects.
3. Drug causes serious adverse reactions including proteinuria and bone marrow depression.
4. Skin rash and loss of taste (dysgeusia) occur frequently. These effects are mild, reversible, and self-limited.
5. Monitoring includes blood pressure, liver function, renal function, and blood cell counts.

PERIPHERAL VASCULAR DISEASES

Peripheral vascular diseases are a group of conditions that involve the veins, arteries, and lymphatic vessels of the extremities. The prevalence of these conditions in older persons, especially those with other chronic health problems, increases with age. While not considered a cause of death, peripheral vascular diseases can be very debilitating. Factors contributing to the development of these vascular problems include arteriosclerosis, atherosclerosis, hyperlipidemia, diabetes mellitus, obesity, hypertension, cardiac conditions, varicose veins, surgery, and prolonged inactivity in any position, including bedrest. These factors may be responsible for a variety of problems, but our discussion will be limited to arteriosclerosis obliterans and thrombophlebitis.

ARTERIOSCLEROSIS OBLITERANS

The signs and symptoms associated with arteriosclerosis obliterans are caused by the ischemia of the tissues nourished by the affected artery. The development and extent of the manifestations depend on the individual's ability to develop adequate collateral circulation.

Signs and symptoms

The most common symptom occurring with arteriosclerosis obliterans is intermittent claudication. The associated pain occurs when the person is walking specific distances; it is relieved by rest and recurs with walking. The pain, which is described as cramping, squeezing, aching, or fatigue, is confined to a specific muscle group. The calf is most commonly affected, but the pain can also occur in the lower back, buttocks, thigh, or foot. As the occlusion progresses, pain may occur at rest, is aggravated by elevation, and is relieved with dependency. Pulses below the area of the occlusion will be diminished or absent. Color changes that can occur include elevation pallor, followed by dependent rubor or cyanosis. Skin and temperature changes that can occur to the feet and legs in serious ischemia include the following: extremities are cool; skin is thin, shiny, and without hair; and nails become thick, brittle, hard, and deformed. If the disease continues to progress, painful ulcers or gangrene can develop.

Management

Management of arteriosclerosis obliterans may be achieved through surgical procedures such as endarterectomy, bypass, graft, or sympathectomy. In more advanced conditions, amputation may be necessary. Health practitioners should focus their interventions on preventing the complications that may occur. A program of prevention should include initiating a graduated walking program, encouraging frequent position change and leg exercises, promoting weight loss if the patient is obese, encouraging cessation of smoking, teaching or providing meticulous foot care, encouraging use of warm socks and avoidance of local heat, teaching correct use of elastic stockings, and providing appropriate care if ulcers are present.

The use of drugs in the management of arterial occlusive vascular disease has met with varying degrees of success. Anticoagulants may be prescribed to prevent future thromboses. Vasodilators, which are sometimes prescribed, seem to have no effect on the diseased vessels.

THROMBOPHLEBITIS

Older persons are more susceptible to thrombophlebitis as a result of pathological vascular changes, extensive surgical procedures, and longer survival of critically ill persons.

Signs and symptoms

Superficial thrombophlebitis is characterized by sudden onset of pain, warmth and redness of the skin over the vein, sensitivity of the area, and edema. The characteristic fever found in younger persons may be absent. If the deep veins are involved, local findings may include edema, cyanosis when standing, and possible positive Homans' sign. The person can feel a heavy, cramplike sensation in the extremity, pain in the sole of the foot, restlessness, and anxiety. The vagueness of the manifestations of deep thrombophlebitis may lead to an incorrect diagnosis, which can result in a serious and sometimes fatal complication, pulmonary embolism.

Management

The primary focus is the prevention of venous thrombosis, which can be practiced at home or in institutional settings. Early ambulation after surgery or acute illness, active or passive exercises for bedfast patients, elevation of extremities, and proper wrapping of the extremities have been demonstrated to be effective in preventing the problem. Superficial thrombophlebitis is treated with heat, rest, elevation of the extremity to enhance venous return, and wrapping the legs with elastic bandages or stockings. A similar but more rigid program is used in treating deep thrombophlebitis.

Anticoagulant therapy may be prescribed before a major surgical procedure and is used to treat deep thrombophlebitis. In the acute-care setting, heparin may be administered followed by warfarin, which may be given for varying lengths of time. Long-term anticoagulation therapy may be indicated.

Anticoagulants: coumarin derivatives
Warfarin

Drug action. Warfarin interferes with liver cell biosynthesis of the plasma precoagulant protein prothrombin and the related clotting factors.

Drug	Dosage
Warfarin sodium	Initial: 10 to 15 mg daily for 2 to 3 days. Maintenance: 2 to 10 mg daily as indicated by prothrombin time determination.

Proper use and precautions
1. Geriatric patients must be closely monitored, because increased anticoagulant effects may occur.
2. Medication is to be taken exactly as prescribed and at the same time each day.
3. A missed dose must be taken as soon as possible and the patient advised to return to the regular schedule.
4. Patients should inform physicians, dentists, nurses, and pharmacists that they are taking this medication.

5. Carrying an identification card and wearing identification indicating that the patient is taking anticoagulants is strongly recommended.
6. Physicians should be consulted before the patient begins or discontinues taking any prescribed or over-the-counter medication because of possible drug interactions.
7. The mechanism of drug interaction is to inhibit or potentiate the action of the anticoagulant. Because of the multiplicity and complexity of drug interactions, refer to Chapter 4.
8. Alcohol intake should be minimized because of its effects on the anticoagulant. Alcohol should be eliminated on a daily basis, and the patient should never exceed two drinks at one time.
9. A normal well-balanced diet should be eaten during the period the medication is taken. No changes in eating habits, particularly in vitamin K-containing foods, should be undertaken without consulting the physician.
10. While the medicine is being taken, the patient should be cautioned not to participate in any activity that may lead to injury. Any blow to the body or other injury should be reported because of the possibility of internal bleeding.
11. The patient should be cautioned to continue the previously described activities 4 to 5 days after treatment is discontinued. At this time the prothrombin level returns to normal.
12. Because of the dangers involved in taking this medication, the practitioner is advised to monitor the regularity of physician visits. While the maintenance dose is being established, the prothrombin time is determined daily. During the maintenance period it is usually measured every 1 to 4 weeks.
13. The antidote for coumarin derivatives is vitamin K (e.g., menadiol sodium diphosphate or phytonadione).
14. Side effects that may occur with the use of warfarin include early signs of overdosage: bleeding from gums when brushing teeth, unusual bleeding or oozing from cuts or wounds, unexplained bruising or purplish areas on skin, and unexplained nosebleeds. Signs of internal bleeding include abdominal pain or swelling, back pain, bloody or tarry stools, bloody or cloudy urine, constipation, coughing up blood, dizziness, severe or continuous headaches, and vomiting blood or coffee-ground–appearing material. Other possible side effects include dark urine, diarrhea, edema of feet and lower legs, itching, skin rash, hives, nausea or vomiting, sore throat, fever, chills, unusual fatigue, sores in mouth or throat, unusual hair loss, and yellowing of eyes.

15. Monitoring includes regular physician visits, signs and symptoms of overdosage, prothrombin time determinations, stool examination for occult blood, and urine examination for blood.

REFERENCE

Kannel, W.B.: Some lessons in cardiovascular epidemiology from Framingham, Am. J. Cardiol. **37:**269, 1976.

SUGGESTED READINGS

Carnavali, D., and Patrick, C.: Nursing management for the elderly, Philadelphia, 1979, J.B. Lippincott Co.

Drayer, J., and Weber, M.: Hypertension in the elderly: a new understanding, Drug Therapy **6:** 91, 1981.

Finnerty, F.: Hypertension in the elderly, Postgrad. Med. **65:**120, 1979.

Haimovici, H.: The peripheral vascular system. In Rossman, I., editor: Clinical geriatrics, Philadelphia, 1979, J.B. Lippincott Co.

Lucas, C.P., and Omar, M.: Pretreatment assessment of the hypertensive patient, Geriatrics **35:**51, 1980.

Moser, M.: Hypertension in the elderly. In Rossman, I., editor: Clinical geriatrics, Philadelphia, 1979, J.B. Lippincott Co.

Niarchos, A., and Laragh, J.: Hypertension in the elderly, Mod. Concepts Cardiovasc. Dis. **49:** 49, 1980.

Ram, C.: Diuretics in the treatment of hypertension, Hospital Formulary **16:**741, 1981.

Rodstein, M.: Heart disease in the aged. In Rossman, I., editor: Clinical geriatrics, Philadelphia, 1979, J.B. Lippincott Co.

Ryan, C.: Guidelines for evaluating and treating hypertension, Geriatrics **34:**43, 1979.

Todd, B.: Drugs and the elderly: when the patient is on diuretics, Geriatr. Nurs. **2:**149, 1981.

12

MANAGEMENT OF SELECTED RESPIRATORY PROBLEMS

As people grow older, they become more vulnerable to viral and bacterial pneumonia, tuberculosis, and chronic obstructive pulmonary disease (COPD), which includes chronic bronchitis, emphysema, and asthma. The reason for this susceptibility is not clear, but factors contributing to it may include anatomical and physiological changes in the lungs, decline in immune function, decrease in mucociliary clearance, and other chronic illnesses. The major focus of this chapter will be on COPD and its related drug therapy. Attention will also be given to pneumonia, a disease that can become serious in older adults, and tuberculosis, which is becoming more common among them.

Because of the susceptibility of older persons to respiratory disease, several measures are recommended to aid in the prevention of pneumonia. Horton and Pankey (1982) suggest that older persons, regardless of their health status, receive pneumococcal vaccine, which prevents pneumonia caused by 14 common pneumococcal types. Booster injections are recommended every 5 years. An annual immunization with influenza vaccine is also recommended for all persons over 65, especially those with COPD, who are particularly vulnerable to influenza. These immunizations should be administered in early fall to give maximum benefit. The medication is effective within 2 to 3 weeks.

CHRONIC OBSTRUCTIVE PULMONARY DISEASE

COPD is a progressive illness that has become increasingly more common in older persons, with men affected more frequently than women. The disease presents a challenge to health practitioners, who must be closely involved with the patient and family as they learn to cope with the disease, medications, equipment, and changing life-style requirements.

A variety of factors contribute to the development of COPD, with cigarette smoking being the most damaging. Under healthy circumstances the airway is cleansed by the action of the cilia, which move the thin layer of mucus upward. Smoking, by paralyzing the cilia, decreases mucociliary clearance. Mucus stasis occurs, the bacteria and other materials are not removed from the airway, and chronic inflammatory changes result. Other factors known to cause COPD include air pollution in heavily industrialized areas, occupations with exposure to dusts and noxious gases, chronic respiratory infections, and hereditary factors. Emphysema may appear at a young age in persons who inherit an antitrypsin deficiency.

COPD includes chronic bronchitis, asthma, and emphysema. A brief discussion of these conditions follows. Chronic bronchitis is characterized by chronic airway inflammation with hypertrophy of tracheobronchial mucous glands. The excretion of excessive mucus production results in a cough. Coughing becomes more difficult with the thickening of the mucus, which in turn interferes with ciliary activity. If the cough and sputum expectoration have been present for at least 3 consecutive months in 2 consecutive years, a diagnosis of chronic bronchitis is made. Other pathological changes that may result in narrowing of the airway and thus interfere with coughing include vasodilatation, congestion, and edema.

Asthma, frequently referred to as a reactive airway disease, is generally a reversible condition, because it is allergenic. The trachea and bronchi are hyperreactive to certain substances. A generalized narrowing of the airway occurs in response to bronchospasm, mucosal edema, and excessive secretion of mucus. With repeated attacks, airway narrowing can become permanent, and lung parenchyma may be thickened and possibly destroyed.

Pulmonary emphysema is an anatomical abnormality characterized by destruction of alveolar walls with distortion and enlargement of the distal area spaces. The end result is a reduction in the area for oxygen and carbon dioxide diffusion and exchange.

Although asthma, chronic bronchitis, and pulmonary emphysema are different pathological entities, most patients with one will usually have another. However, the degree of involvement ranges from chronic bronchitis with no emphysema through various combinations to severe emphysema with significant bronchitis (Sexton, 1981).

COPD, which includes chronic bronchitis, asthma, and pulmonary emphysema, is now the sixth leading cause of death in this country. A potentially incapacitating illness, COPD is a major health problem.

Signs and symptoms

The two major symptoms of the person with COPD are shortness of breath and cough. The shortness of breath, which is increased by physical activity, is frequently accompanied by wheezing and prolonged expiration, which are caused by obstruction of air flow. Collapsed airways, excessive mucus, and bronchospasm may be responsible for this interference. The cough, which may be precipitated by a change in position, may result in expectoration of sputum varying from small amounts of thick mucus to copious amounts of mucopurulent material. Sputum is generally most abundant when the person arises in the morning. These symptoms may be accompanied by the characteristic barrel chest with an increase in anteroposterior diameter, which suggests hyperinflation of the lungs. However, this variation in shape is due in part to the normal aging process. As the disease progresses, the patient has weight loss, tachycardia, and rapid breathing with any exertion. Cyanosis may be present.

Management

The chronicity and progressiveness of COPD necessitate an individualized treatment plan formulated by various health disciplines with input by the patient and family members. The objectives of management include maintenance of function at an optimum level, prevention of complications, rehabilitation, control of symptoms, and patient education. To achieve these goals, the program should include the following components: coughing and breathing, airway management, use of oxygen and breathing equipment, appropriate living environment, nutrition and hydration, physical conditioning, and drug management. We recognize the importance of all program components, but our discussion is limited to drug management.

Patients with COPD receive a variety of medications to control the symptoms of the disease. These drugs, which include bronchodilators, steroids, and antibiotics, are most effective for persons with reversible airway diseases such as asthma and bronchitis.

Bronchodilators

Bronchodilators, the cornerstone of drug therapy, fall into three main classes, the β-adrenergic agents, the methylxanthines, and the anticholinergics. Each class of drugs acts in a different way and has its own disadvantages.

The action of the first class of drugs, the β-adrenergic agents, is mediated through β_1 and β_2 receptors, each of which has a different function. When the β_1 receptors are stimulated, the heart is affected by increased force of contraction (inotropic effect) and increased heart rate (chronotropic effect). Stimulation of the β_2 receptors causes relaxation of the smooth muscles of the tracheobronchial tree.

Unfortunately, all β-adrenergic drugs have a stimulatory effect on both the β_1 and β_2 receptors, but in the more recently developed drugs, the β_2 effects exceed the β_1 effects, and this difference results in greater influence on the tracheobronchial tree and less stimulation of the heart. Metaproterenol sulfate, terbutaline sulfate, albuterol sulfate, and isoetharine are drugs exhibiting these effects.

All β-adrenergic bronchodilators are capable of stimulating the cardiovascular system, which may already be weakened through the aging process or pathological changes. In older persons these drugs must be used in smaller doses and used with caution in the presence of angina and arrhythmias. Close observation is essential.

β-Adrenergic bronchodilators can be administered orally or parenterally or by aerosol. Aerosol administration is the preferred route for treatment of acute attacks. The aerosol can be delivered by a variety of devices ranging from the hand-held to the power-driven nebulizers to the intermittent positive pressure breathing devices. When using the β-adrenergic bronchodilators, patients should be cautioned to use the aerosol medications only on a scheduled basis, since tolerance readily develops.

The second group of bronchodilators, the methylxanthines, act by inhibiting the enzyme phosphodiesterase, which results in impaired breakdown of adenosine monophosphate (cyclic AMP). The methylxanthines may be used separately but may also be used in conjunction with another bronchodilator. Since the difference between the therapeutic and toxic dose is small, serum levels must be monitored to prevent serious side effects. Major side effects are seizures and supraventricular tachycardia, and minor effects include nausea, vomiting, headache, nervousness, and agitation.

Oral preparations of the methylxanthines are available and should be used around-the-clock to prevent wheezing and other problems common to patients with COPD. The longer-acting methylxanthines with effects lasting 8 to 12 hours have proved effective. Fixed combinations of drugs have not proved as successful as the administration of individual agents, since only one of the drugs may be an offender in the development of side effects or toxicity.

Anticholinergics, the third class of bronchodilators, block cholinergic stimulation and decrease intracellular guanosine monophosphate (cyclic GMP). Newer atropine-like agents (e.g., ipratropium bromide) with decreased side effects may soon be released, and their availability will decrease the disadvantages of currently available drugs.

β-Adrenergic agents

Drug action. β-Adrenergic agents produce bronchodilation by causing relaxation of smooth muscle in bronchi.

Drug	Availability	Dosage
Isoetharine	Metered solution (0.61%)	One to three inhalations q.4-6h.
	Inhalant solution (1%)	Three to four inhalations q.4-6h.
Metaproterenol	Oral	20 mg q.6-8h.
	Metered powder	Two to three inhalations q.4-8h.
	Inhalant solution (5%)	Four to ten inhalations q.4-8h.
Terbutaline	Oral	Avoid if possible because of cardiovascular side effects.
	Subcutaneous	0.125 to 0.25 mg q.4h.
Albuterol	Metered inhalant	Two inhalations q.4-6h.
	Oral	2 mg t.i.d. or q.i.d. with gradual increase if needed.

Proper use and precautions
1. The medications are to be used only as directed.
2. The medications are administered by different methods; therefore instructions must be followed carefully.
3. If the patient has difficulty breathing after using the medication, the physician should be notified immediately.
4. Drug interactions may occur with propranolol (may antagonize bronchodilative effects) and sympathomimetics (may increase effects of either medication and their potential side effects).
5. Side effects that may occur are related to sympathomimetic actions and include dizziness, light-headedness, headache, nausea, nervousness, restlessness, insomnia, weakness, unusually fast or pounding heartbeat, chest pain, and trembling.
6. Monitoring includes regular physician visits, signs and symptoms of overdosage, cardiac function, blood glucose (for diabetic patients), and aerosol tachyphylaxis.

Methylxanthines: theophylline and theophylline ethylenediamine (aminophylline)

Drug action. By inhibiting the action of phosphodiesterase, the methylxanthines catalyze the breakdown of cyclic AMP.

Drug	Dosage
Aminophylline	Maintenance: 7 to 14 mg/kg/day.
Theophylline	Maintenance: 6 to 12 mg/kg/day.

Optimum serum concentration is between 10 and 20 μg/ml.

Proper use and precautions
1. The medication should be taken with a full glass of water either 30 to 60 minutes before a meal or 2 hours after a meal for faster absorption. However, it can be taken with meals if gastric irritation is a problem.
2. Dosages are very individualized, and monitoring of serum theophyl-

line levels is required because of the very narrow therapeutic range. Dosage is decreased in congestive heart failure and liver disease.
3. Dosages for geriatric patients are less, because theophylline clearance is generally decreased.
4. Smoking increases the metabolism of theophylline and consequently affects dosage.
5. Caffeine-containing beverages—coffee, tea, cocoa, and cola—should be avoided, since they may increase the CNS stimulation effects of the drug.
6. Drug interactions may occur with erythromycin (may decrease theophylline clearance, resulting in increased serum levels with the danger of toxicity), cimetidine (may increase serum theophylline levels), lithium (renal excretion of lithium is increased, lowering therapeutic levels), propranolol (effects of both drugs may be decreased), and other methylxanthine derivatives (may increase danger of toxicity).
7. Side effects that indicate symptoms of toxicity include bloody or tarry stools, cloudy urine, increased urination, muscle twitching, confusion, seizures, vomiting blood (red or dark brown), unusual thirst, fatigue, and fast and bounding pulse. Other effects may include skin rash or hives, anorexia, nausea, vomiting, stomach pain, diarrhea, headache, nervousness, irritability, dizziness, insomnia, flushing of face, and unusually rapid breathing.
8. Monitoring includes regular physician visits, pulmonary function measurements, and serum theophylline levels.

Steroids

The use of antiinflammatory steroids in lung disease has been found to be most successful in asthma. Wynne (1979) lists the following conditions in which patients may benefit from the use of steroids: wheezing, marked response to β-adrenergic bronchodilators, history of allergies, and sputum or blood eosinophilia.

Because of the side effects to which older persons are especially vulnerable, a short course of therapy, in which side effects occur less frequently, may be the treatment of choice. Prednisone, 5 to 60 mg daily, will generally bring relief of symptoms. Administration of the drug on alternate days has proved to cause less adrenal suppression than administering the drug in smaller divided daily doses. However, alternate-day therapy is often not tolerated by the patient, because symptoms return on the drug-free day. Steroids are available in oral, intramuscular, intravenous, and inhalation forms.

The development of a surface active topical corticosteroid, beclomethasone, was a major advance for patients with lung disease. The drug is inhaled directly into the lungs and has fewer side effects than systemic steroids do. However, localized *Candida* infections have occurred in the mouth and pharynx as a result of beclomethasone therapy. This drug is used with caution for older people because of the risk of adrenal insufficiency during and following transfer from systemic corticosteroids to the aerosol route of administration.

Prednisone

Drug action. Prednisone inhibits the inflammatory response.

Drug	Dosage
Prednisone	5 to 60 mg daily.

Proper use and precautions
1. Medication is to be taken only as directed and not discontinued without consultation with the physician.
2. Medication may be taken with food to minimize stomach upset.
3. Alcohol should be avoided, because it can increase ulcerogenic effects.
4. With long-term therapy, an alternate-day regimen is suggested to minimize hypothalamic-pituitary-adrenal suppression.
5. Dietary alterations that may be necessary include low sodium, high potassium, or decreased calories.
6. The physician should be advised that the patient is taking this medication in the following circumstances: before having a vaccination, immunization, or skin test; before having any type of surgery; and if a serious infection or injury occurs.
7. Diabetic patients should be advised that this drug may cause an elevation in blood glucose level.
8. Drug interactions that may occur include alcohol or antiinflammatory drugs (increase ulcerogenic effects), potassium-depleting diuretics (may increase arrhythmias or digitalis toxicity), coumarin-type anticoagulants (may affect dosage requirements), hypoglycemics (may increase blood glucose levels, requiring dosage adjustments), and salicylates (lower plasma concentration of salicylates may occur); salicylism may occur after steroid dosage is decreased or discontinued.
9. Drug interferes with many diagnostic studies.
10. Side effects that may occur include blurred vision, frequent urination, increased thirst, or skin rash (require medical intervention); skin problems, back or rib pain, bloody or tarry stools, stomach pain,

mood changes, susceptibility to infections, irregular heartbeat, muscle cramps or weakness or pain, unusual fatigue, nausea or vomiting, moon face, weight gain, edema, seeing halos around lights, nervousness, and insomnia.
11. Monitoring includes regular physician visits; blood, glucose, and electrolyte determinations; stool examination for occult blood; and ophthalmic examination (if therapy extends beyond 6 weeks).

Beclomethasone

Drug action. Beclomethasone inhibits the inflammatory response.

Drug	Dosage
Beclomethasone dipropionate	Two inhalations (84 μg) three to four times daily. Maximum should not exceed 20 inhalations.

Proper use and precautions
1. Beclomethasone is administered in a metered-dose aerosol unit that delivers 42 μg/inhalation.
2. The medication is used on a regular basis for prophylactic therapy as prescribed by the physician. One to four weeks may pass before full effect is noticed.
3. Drug is used with caution if bacterial, fungal, or viral infection of the mouth, throat, or lungs exists.
4. Use is contraindicated for patients sensitive to fluorocarbon propellants or other aerosol spray medications.
5. Gargling and rinsing the mouth after each dose will help prevent hoarseness and throat irritation.
6. Patients receiving systemic steroids should continue to take both medications until a program of gradual withdrawal of the oral steroid is prescribed by the physician.
7. A concurrently prescribed bronchodilator inhaler should be used several minutes before the beclomethasone inhaler to enhance the penetration of the steroid into the bronchial tree.
8. Monitoring includes regular physician visits, signs of mouth or throat infection, and aerosol tachyphylaxis.

PNEUMONIA

Older adults are especially susceptible to pneumonia because of the aging changes that take place in the lungs, the probable decline of the immune system, and the presence of chronic illness, particularly COPD. Pneumococcal pneumonia is the most commonly occurring type in older people. Because the illness presents an atypical picture, the diagnosis is frequently missed, and as a result pneumonia remains a major cause of death in older persons.

Signs and symptoms

The usual signs of pneumonia found in younger persons, the cough, fever, purulent sputum, and chest pain, may be mild or absent; instead there may be more subtle symptoms such as anorexia, lethargy, tachypnea, and tachycardia (Wynne, 1979).

Management

Before beginning therapy a bacteriological examination of the sputum and a Gram stain should be done. The identification of the specific infecting agent determines the choice of antibiotic therapy. For critically ill elderly patients a broad-spectrum antibiotic should be administered to cover suspected organisms before the identification of the specific organism.

In addition to the drug management with antimicrobial therapy, supportive therapy is required. Bedrest, adequate hydration, postural drainage, use of oxygen, and prevention of recurrence are important components of care.

Pneumonia is most commonly caused by a gram-positive coccus. The drug of choice is penicillin. Erythromycin or a cephalosporin derivative can be used if the patient is allergic to penicillin or if the organism is resistant to penicillin.

Antibiotics

Antibiotics are used to treat respiratory infections that may progress to pneumonia and other exacerbations of COPD. Patients should be alerted to signs and symptoms that may indicate a respiratory infection and to initiate treatment immediately. Symptoms include increased cough and sputum production, thickening of the sputum, which becomes yellow, green, or gray in color, increased shortness of breath, feeling of tightness in chest, and fever or chills.

Because of the urgency for treatment and the unpredictability of the tracheal flora in patients with COPD, cultures may be omitted. Some patients receive prophylactic therapy throughout the year or during the winter months when susceptibility to infection increases. As with other antibiotic therapy, a full course of 7 to 20 days must be completed to be effective.

TUBERCULOSIS

The pattern of tuberculosis has changed over the past years. The number of cases of active tuberculosis in younger persons has markedly decreased as a result of effective antituberculosis therapy. However, active tuberculosis is occurring more frequently in older persons, in persons previously affected, and in those with increased susceptibility. Persons who are particularly vulnerable include those with chronic illnesses such as diabetes and silicosis, persons receiving immunosuppressive therapy, and those who have poor nutrition. These chronic conditions, when complicated by tuberculosis, are responsible for high death rates.

Signs and symptoms

The typical characteristics of tuberculosis are fever, night sweats, weight loss, fatigue, productive cough, hemoptysis, and chest pain. However, since the older person may present an atypical picture with nonspecific vague symptoms, the disease may be missed until it has reached advanced stages. Radiological findings are also atypical. In addition to these atypical characteristics, the diagnosis may be missed because of anergy to purified protein derivative (PPD). The change in tuberculin sensitivity increases after the age of 70 (Wynne, 1979).

Management

Before considering conventional drug therapy used in the treatment of tuberculosis, attention will be given to prevention of the active disease. Persons who have a positive reaction to PPD are candidates for a 1-year course of therapy of isoniazid, 300 mg daily. However, the possibility of developing serious side effects such as hepatitis to isoniazid therapy increases in older persons, and unless there are additional risk factors predisposing the patient, preventive treatment may be withheld. Factors indicating the need for treatment include recent conversion to positive PPD response and the presence of household contacts. Because of the hepatic complications, close monitoring of persons receiving isoniazid prophylactically is essential.

In older persons, early recognition of the disease and initiation of therapy are important. Because the older person is very sensitive to side effects of the drugs, Wynne (1979) recommends a conservative approach to therapy. He and others (Estepan and King, 1981) suggest a two-drug approach. Despite its side effects, isoniazid is still considered a first-line drug and is included in initial treatment. Ethambutol is the second most commonly used drug, with rifampin reserved for more resistant-type disease in which a third drug may be indicated. Streptomycin has limited use for older persons, because toxicity develops earlier in this group and the effects on the eighth cranial nerve are not well tolerated.

Antituberculosis drugs
Isoniazid

Drug action. Isoniazid acts against actively growing tubercle bacilli.

Drug	Dosage
Isoniazid	Prophylactic: 300 mg daily.
	Therapeutic: 5 mg/kg of body weight, up to 300 mg daily.

Proper use and precautions
1. Medication may be taken in single or divided doses with food to prevent gastric upset.
2. Smaller doses of isoniazid are recommended for persons with impaired hepatic function.
3. A full course of therapy, which may take 1 to 2 years, is essential to produce a cure.
4. Vitamin B_6 (pyridoxine), 50 to 100 mg daily, may be prescribed concurrently to decrease the incidence of peripheral neuritis.
5. Alcohol must be avoided, because it increases the danger of liver damage and decreases the effectiveness of the medication.
6. Diabetic patients should be cautioned that the drug may cause false-positive test results with copper sulfate urine glucose tests.
7. Patients should be cautioned about the prodromal signs of hepatitis (such as fever and malaise) or peripheral neuritis (burning, tingling, and numbness), which should be reported to the physician immediately.
8. Drug interactions that may occur include alcohol (increases danger of hepatotoxicity and increased metabolism of isoniazid), aluminum- and magnesium-containing antacids (may delay and decrease absorption and serum levels of isoniazid), disulfiram (may increase CNS effects of disulfiram), phenytoin (may increase phenytoin serum levels and toxicity), and rifampin (increases risk of hepatotoxicity).
9. Side effects that require prompt medical attention include unusual weakness or tiredness; clumsiness or unsteadiness; numbness, tingling, burning, or pain in hands and feet; nausea; vomiting; yellowing of skin or eyes; and blurring or loss of vision with or without eye pain. Other side effects include dizziness, upset stomach, and enlarged breasts.
10. Monitoring includes regular physician visits, hepatic function determinations (serum glutamic-oxaloacetic transaminase [SGOT] or serum glutamic-pyruvic transaminase [SGPT]) at regular intervals,

close monitoring of side effects, and ophthalmoscopic examination if visual symptoms occur.

Ethambutol

Drug action. Ethambutol is tuberculostatic and is used in combination with other tuberculostatic drugs in treating tuberculosis. It is effective only against mycobacteria.

Drug	Dosage
Ethambutol (in combination with other tuberculostatic drugs)	Initial treatment: 15 mg/kg of body weight daily. Retreatment: 25 mg/kg of body weight daily for 60 to 90 days; then 15 mg/kg of body weight daily.

Proper use and precautions
1. Medication may be taken with food to prevent gastric upset.
2. Drug should be taken in a single daily dose to reach effective serum levels.
3. A full course of therapy, which may take 1 to 2 years, is essential to produce a cure.
4. Drug must be administered concurrently with other tuberculostatics, because bacterial resistance may develop rapidly when it is administered alone.
5. Older adults with impaired renal function may require a smaller dose.
6. Drug may cause elevations in serum uric acid levels, possibly precipitating gout.
7. Visual changes (visual field, visual acuity, and color discrimination) may occur.
8. Drug interactions are not documented.
9. Side effects that require prompt medical attention include blurred vision or any loss of vision, eye pain, or red-green color blindness; chills, pain, and swelling over joints (especially great toe, ankle, or knee); or tense hot skin over affected joints. Other side effects that may occur include numbness, tingling, or burning of hands or feet; dizziness; itching; rash; or stomach upset.
10. Monitoring includes regular physician visits, serum uric acid determinations, and ophthalmoscopic examination (visual fields and acuity, red-green color discrimination) with doses over 15 mg/kg of body weight daily.

Rifampin

Drug action. Rifampin is a tuberculostatic drug used in combination with other tuberculostatic drugs in treating tuberculosis; it is also used to treat asymptomatic meningococcal carriers by eliminating *Neisseria meningitidis* from the nasopharynx.

Drug	Dosage
Rifampin	Elderly and debilitated patients: 10 mg/kg of body weight daily. Usual adult dose: 600 mg daily (in combination with other tuberculostatic drugs).

Proper use and precautions

1. Rifampin should be taken with a full glass of water on an empty stomach (1 hour before or 2 hours after a meal) to achieve optimum absorption. If gastric distress occurs, the medication can be taken with meals.
2. A full course of therapy, which may take 1 to 2 years, is essential to produce a cure.
3. Alcohol must be avoided, because it increases danger of liver damage and decreases the effectiveness of rifampin.
4. Smaller dosages are required for persons with impaired hepatic function (not to exceed 8 mg/kg of body weight daily).
5. Drug must be administered concurrently with other tuberculostatic drugs, because bacterial resistance may occur rapidly when rifampin is administered alone.
6. Medication may cause urine, feces, saliva, sputum, sweat, and tears to turn orange to reddish brown.
7. Soft contact lenses may become discolored.
8. Drug interferes with many diagnostic studies.
9. Drug interactions that may occur include alcohol (may increase danger of hepatotoxicity and increase metabolism of rifampin), oral anticoagulants, corticosteroids, digitoxin, tolbutamide (their effects may be decreased), isoniazid (may increase danger of hepatotoxicity), methadone (may decrease effects of methadone), and probenecid (may cause increased or prolonged rifampin levels).
10. Side effects that require prompt medical attention include chills, shivering, breathing problems, dizziness, fever, headache, and muscle or bone pain; decreased frequency of urination and decreased amount of urine; loss of appetite, nausea, and vomiting; unusual fatigue or weakness; yellowing of eyes or skin; and unusual bleeding or bruising. Other side effects that may occur include stomach cramps; diarrhea; discolored urine, feces, saliva, sputum, sweat, and tears; itching; rash; redness; and sore mouth or tongue.
11. Monitoring includes regular physician visits, hepatic function determination (SGOT or SGPT) at regular intervals, and close monitoring of side effects.

REFERENCES

Estepan, H., and King, T.: Treating respiratory diseases in the elderly, Drug Therapy **6:**55, 1981.

Horton, J., and Pankey, G.: Pneumonia in the elderly, Postgrad. Med. **71:**114, 1982.

Sexton, D.L.: Chronic obstructive pulmonary disease: care of the child and adult, St. Louis, 1981, The C.V. Mosby Co.

Wynne, J.: Pulmonary diseases in the elderly. In Rossman, I., editor: Clinical geriatrics, ed. 2, Philadelphia, 1979, J.B. Lippincott Co.

SUGGESTED READINGS

Carnevali, D., and Patrick, M.: Nursing management for the elderly, Philadelphia, 1979, J.B. Lippincott Co.

Futrell, M., and others: Primary health care of the older adult, North Scituate, Mass., 1980, Duxbury Press.

Mathers, J., and others: Office management of COPD, Geriatrics **36:**103, 1981.

Pierson, D., and Leonard, L.: Evaluation of dyspnea, Geriatrics **36:**48, 1981.

Stanezak, W.: Case studies in pharmacy practice, U.S. Pharmacist **6:**25, 1981.

Ziment, I.: How to select an appropriate respiratory drug, Geriatrics **36:**89, 1981.

13

MANAGEMENT OF SELECTED GASTROINTESTINAL PROBLEMS

Symptoms of gastrointestinal dysfunction are common in older persons. The complaints are frequently vague and may be atypical when compared with those of younger persons. The more commonly occurring problems and related therapy reviewed in this chapter include peptic ulcers, constipation, and diarrhea. Each of these disorders can have serious effects.

PEPTIC ULCERS

The incidence of peptic ulcers has shown an increase that may relate to the stress placed on older persons. The stress caused by sudden illness or emotional trauma is known to precipitate peptic ulcers. The side effects of various medications such as salicylates and corticosteroids are known to increase the rate of ulcer formation.

Signs and symptoms

The characteristic epigastric pain found in younger persons with peptic ulcers may be absent in older persons. As with many illnesses that strike older adults, the symptoms may be vague. The patient may complain of generalized abdominal pain, lack of appetite, vomiting, loss of weight, and low energy levels. Bleeding may be absent until an acute perforation of the ulcer occurs.

Management

Earlier methods of treating peptic ulcers with half-and-half or whole milk are no longer used, because milk and cream were found to have a rebound acid effect. The use of skim or low-fat milk is advised. Caffeine, spices, and smoking should be avoided because of gastric stimulatory effects. Patients

TABLE 8. Gastric antacids

Drug name	Dosage	Comments
Aluminum compounds		
Aluminum hydroxide gel	5-40 ml 2 tablets, 5-6 times daily (well chewed)	Low neutralizing capacity; given in conjunction with milk to prevent constipation; may bind dietary phosphatase in bowel, leading to osteoporosis or osteomalacia; unbound dietary calcium may result in elevated blood and urine levels, leading to stone formation in renal tissue.
Calcium compounds		
Calcium carbonate, precipitated	5-15 ml 2 or more tablets	Potent, rapid, and relatively prolonged acid-neutralizing effect. Causes constipation; best if administered with magnesium compounds; contraindicated if there is history of kidney stones.
Magnesium compounds		
Milk of magnesia	5-30 ml, 4 or more times daily 2-4 tablets, 4 times daily	Prompt and effective neutralizer of gastric acid with relatively prolonged action; in dosages adequate (15-30 ml) for intensive therapy, diarrhea may result; combined with calcium carbonate or aluminum hydroxide, reduces laxative effect; in older adults with severe renal impairment, systemic absorption of magnesium may occur.
Combinations of aluminum and magnesium compounds		
Magnesium and aluminum oral suspension	5-30 ml 2-4 tablets (well chewed)	Neutralizing power of magnesium and acid-binding capacity of aluminum provide reliable reaction.

frequently need counseling about alterations in life-style that are necessary to relieve the stress that may have caused the ulcer.

Antacid therapy

The most prevalent use of antacids is in the management of peptic ulcers. However, since antacids are available without prescription, they are used for hyperacidity symptoms ascribed to acid indigestion, heartburn, sour or upset stomach, full feeling, belching, and overeating. Because of the availability for self-administration, the pharmacist or nurse may be called on to recommend a particular product.

The criteria used in the selection of an ideal antacid are the following: it neutralizes gastric acid, has a prolonged action, is not absorbed from the gastrointestinal tract, has minimum amount of sodium, does not cause constipation or diarrhea, does not affect the pH or electrolyte balance, has no acid rebound, and is not reactive to other drugs in the gastrointestinal tract (Wuest and Gossel, 1981).

Factors to consider in making an antacid recommendation are the adverse effects that are possible with each of them. The older adult with renal impairment may absorb antacid ingredient ions, which can produce systemic or urinary alkalosis. Constipation caused by aluminum-containing preparations and diarrhea caused by magnesium preparations are side effects that may result in noncompliance.

The most commonly used antacids are calcium carbonate, magnesium hydroxide, and aluminum hydroxide. Liquid antacids have a buffering capacity that is superior to solid preparations. The advantages and disadvantages of the medications in these categories can be found in Table 8.

Proper use and precautions

1. Medication should be taken at the prescribed time as a means of preventing the pain associated with ulcers. A dose of antacid 1 to 3 hours after meals will generally relieve the pain that occurs when the stomach empties 1½ hours after eating. A bedtime dose will counteract the high acidity occurring between 11 PM and 3 AM.
2. The dosage of an antacid will vary from person to person according to the amount of acid secreted.
3. Tablets need to be thoroughly chewed and followed by water for optimum effectiveness.
4. Patients with renal impairment, congestive heart failure, edema, and hypertension should be monitored when requiring chronic antacid therapy because of salt load.
5. Patients on salt-restricted diets require careful monitoring and the use of a low-sodium antacid.
6. Significant side effects of antacid therapy:

Antacid	Constipation	Diarrhea	Acid rebound	Hypermagnesemia	Hypophosphatemia	Hypernatremia	Alkalosis
Sodium bicarbonate			X			X	X
Aluminum hydroxide	X				X		
Magnesium hydroxide		X		X			
Calcium carbonate			X				

7. Interactions with many drugs occur with concurrent antacid therapy because of gastric alkalinization (e.g., quinidine), change in the gastric emptying time (e.g., salicylates), increased binding (e.g., digoxin), and the capacity to form complexes that decrease drug bioavailability (e.g., tetracyclines, iron, benzodiazepines, and phenothiazines).
8. Monitoring includes symptoms of constipation and diarrhea and plasma magnesium, calcium, and aluminum levels in patients with severe renal impairment.

Drugs that reduce gastric acid secretion are also useful in treating peptic and duodenal ulcers in older persons. Cimetidine, a histamine H_2-receptor antagonist, and the anticholinergic propantheline will be discussed.

Histamine H_2-receptor antagonist
Cimetidine

Drug action. Cimetidine blocks the action of histamine at receptors in the acid-secreting parietal cells of the gastric mucosal glands. By reducing the basal gastric acid secretion, the drug has been effective for relief of pain and promotion of healing of duodenal ulcers. Cimetidine has been found to interact with a number of drugs because of several mechanisms of action. Cimetidine inhibits drug-metabolizing enzymes in the liver. It also may reduce hepatic blood flow, which may reduce the first-pass metabolism of drugs such as propranolol. By increasing the pH in the stomach, cimetidine may increase the bioavailability of drugs unstable in acid and alter absorption of other drugs. It has also been suggested that cimetidine may increase the possibility of bone marrow suppression if used concurrently with other drugs capable of depressing bone marrow function.

Drug	Dosage
Cimetidine	Duodenal ulcers: 200 to 300 mg two to four times daily. Hypersecretory conditions: 300 mg four times daily.

Proper use and precautions
1. Older adults with impaired renal function need reduced dosages, beginning with 300 mg every 12 hours and increasing the dose to 300 mg every 8 hours if there are no ill effects.
2. The medication is taken with meals and at bedtime.
3. Antacids may be required early in the course of treatment, because the pain-relieving effects of cimetidine may not be immediately effective.
4. Coumarin anticoagulants given concurrently with cimetidine increase the risk of hypothrombinemia.
5. Side effects that may occur include mental confusion (especially in older adults), diarrhea, dizziness, headaches, muscle cramps or pain, skin rash, and swelling or soreness of breasts.
6. Drug interactions: see Chapter 4.
7. Monitoring includes regular physician visits and evaluating effectiveness of altered doses.

Anticholinergics
Propantheline

Drug action. Propantheline acts centrally by blocking the central synaptic transmission in cholinergic nerve pathways. The drug is used primarily as an antispasmodic-antisecretory agent for patients with peptic ulcer, pancreatitis, and gastritis.

Drug	Dosage
Propantheline bromide tablets	15 mg three times daily; 30 mg at bedtime.
Propantheline bromide extended-release tablets	30 mg every 12 hours.

Proper use and precautions
1. Geriatric patients and persons of less than normal body weight may require one half the usual recommended dose. Response to the usual adult dose may include excitement, agitation, confusion, and drowsiness.
2. The medication is taken ½ to 1 hour before meals.
3. Antacids and antidiarrheals should not be taken within 1 hour of taking this medication.
4. The medication may cause drowsiness; therefore patients should be cautioned about operating an automobile or mechanical appliances.
5. Patients should be cautioned to avoid overheating through exercise in hot weather.
6. Visual sensitivity to light may occur. The use of sunglasses is recommended.
7. Sugarless gum, ice, or sugarless hard candy will help to relieve the

dry mouth caused by the drug. A regular program of oral hygiene and the use of artificial saliva can also provide relief.

8. Constipation should be reported to the physician.

9. Drug interactions that may occur include alcohol or other CNS depressants (may increase sedative effects), amantadine, antimuscarinics, MAO inhibitors, phenothiazine, procainamide, quinidine, tricyclic antidepressants (atropine-like effects intensified), antacids, or antidiarrheal suspensions (may reduce therapeutic effects of propantheline).

10. Side effects that may occur include constipation, difficult urination, eye pain and skin rash, bloated feeling, dry mouth, dizziness, headache, rapid pulse, decreased sweating, blurred vision, increased sensitivity to light, nervousness, tiredness, drowsiness, mental confusion (especially in the elderly), impotence, decreased sense of taste, nausea, and vomiting.

11. Monitoring includes regular physician visits and measurement of intraocular pressure.

CONSTIPATION

Complaints about constipation by an elderly person may revolve around misconceptions about normal bowel function and do not necessarily imply actual constipation. Constipation is defined as a decrease in the frequency of bowel movements accompanied by prolonged and difficult passage of stool, followed by a sensation of incomplete evacuation.

The belief that a person must have a daily bowel movement is commonly held by both the young and old in our society. Bowel patterns in older persons may undergo changes as aging occurs. This alteration is attributed to several factors: inadequate bulk in the diet, inadequate fluid intake, lack of physical exercise, depression, medications, and changes in the gastrointestinal tract. Assessing the changes that have occurred in the person's life will frequently reveal problems that can be resolved without the use of laxatives.

Signs and symptoms

Complaints of constipation from older persons should be investigated. Areas that need further assessment include a description of normal bowel patterns, appearance and frequency of evacuation, recent changes in diet, fluid intake, activity, medication, and stress. If possible, the stool should be observed. Signs and symptoms that may accompany constipation include headache, irritability, lack of appetite, nausea, abdominal cramps, active gas pattern, abdominal distention, absence of bowel movement for a period of time, and fecal incontinence.

Management

Prevention of constipation by diet, hydration, and exercise should be part of the health program for the older adult population. Of equal importance is allowing the person the time, space, and privacy to maintain a consistent pattern of bowel elimination. Maintaining a daily fluid intake of 2000 to 3000 ml of a variety of liquids, unless contraindicated by another condition, also promotes regular bowel habits. A well-balanced diet of fresh fruits and vegetables, whole-grain products, bran, and other high-fiber foods is part of a preventive program. A daily program of exercise that promotes overall body functioning should be part of the total plan in preventing constipation.

When constipation does occur, the preceding measures should still be implemented, but the addition of oral laxatives, suppositories, or enemas may become part of the program.

Laxatives are the single most commonly used medications in nursing homes and skilled nursing facilities, with approximately 60% of the patients receiving one laxative daily (Lamy, 1979). Because laxatives are available without prescription, it is difficult to determine the number and quantity taken by ambulatory older persons.

Laxative use must be clearly evaluated, because valid indications are limited. For persons who must avoid straining because of cardiovascular and cerebral pathophysiological changes, who have marked gastrointestinal changes, or who have altered motility because of prescribed drugs and dietary intake, laxatives may be indicated. According to the need, laxatives can be selected from the following groups: stimulants, saline types, stool softeners, and bulk producers.

Laxatives recommended for older adults
Stimulants

Drug action. Stimulants initiate peristalsis by local irritation of the intestinal wall or by action exerted on intestinal nerves or muscle.

Drug	Dosage
Bisacodyl	10 mg.
Danthron	75 to 150 mg.

Bulk producers

Drug action. Bulk producers stimulate peristalsis by forming a bulky jellylike mass in the intestines.

Drug	Dosage
Psyllium hydrophilic mucilloid	4 to 10 gm.

Stool softeners

Drug action. Stool softeners reduce surface tension of fecal contents of rectum, allowing water to penetrate and produce a bulky mass.

Drug	Dosage
Docusate calcium	50 to 240 mg.
Docusate sodium	50 to 100 mg.

Saline types

Drug action. Saline types attract water to the intestinal lumen, where water is retained, creating intestinal motility.

Drug	Dosage
Milk of magnesia	15 to 30 ml.

Proper use and precautions

1. Patients should be advised that intake of adequate fiber in the form of fruits, vegetables, and grains, intake of adequate fluids, and a regular program of exercise should be part of a daily health program, with or without the use of laxatives.
2. Laxative dependency may occur with habitual use.
3. Drug interactions that may occur are not clinically significant except that milk of magnesia decreases tetracycline absorption, docusate sodium decreases mineral oil absorption, mineral oil causes variations in effects of anticoagulants, and prolonged administration of mineral oil reduces absorption of fat-soluble vitamins (A, D, E, and K).
4. Side effects that may occur include nausea, cramping, diarrhea, and electrolyte imbalance.

DIARRHEA

Diarrhea in an older person is a potentially serious problem because of the limited ability to tolerate fluid and electrolyte loss. Excessive fluid and electrolyte depletion becomes a serious threat to the person's health. For this reason, it is urgent that the cause of the diarrhea be investigated and eliminated if possible. Medication-induced diarrhea is a side effect that occurs more commonly in older than in younger persons. Among the drugs that may be responsible for diarrhea are broad-spectrum antibiotics, colchicine, ferrous sulfate, guanethidine, magnesium-containing antacids, quinidine, griseofulvin, and bethanechol. If patients are aware of this possible side effect of medications, they can report the response to the physician, who can make necessary changes in therapy. Additional factors responsible for diarrhea include emotional stress, intestinal infections, malignant tumors, muscular weakness, neurological problems, and fecal impaction. The diarrhea associated with fecal impaction is more commonly called fecal incontinence.

Signs and symptoms

The signs and symptoms of diarrhea include frequent, watery stools that may be accompanied by abdominal cramping. Stool color varies, and a greenish color generally indicates rapid movement through the small intestines. Mucus or blood may accompany the diarrhea. Because dehydration may rapidly occur, older persons must be carefully observed both for this condition and for possible potassium or sodium depletion. Manifestations of potassium loss include apathy, malaise, general weakness, lassitude, and cardiac arrhythmias. Sodium loss may be exhibited by loss of skin turgor, brownish tongue, sunken cheeks, thirst, and orthostatic hypotension. In prolonged sodium and potassium depletion, other serious complications may occur.

Management

Before establishing a management program, a brief history should be taken to investigate the prescribed or over-the-counter medications being taken, foods recently eaten, stress, and a history of bowel patterns. This history is useful to the practitioner, who may suggest referral to the physician who can get at the source of the problem. However, the nurse can identify and possibly remove the fecal impaction, preferably by removing the stool and then administering a warm oil-retention enema, allowing time for the patient to expel the hard stool, and following the procedure with a soap-suds enema. Other factors to consider in the general management of diarrhea include prompt fluid replacement, protection against dehydration from further fluid loss, and providing a nonirritating diet. Electrolyte supplement solutions such as Gatorade are recommended.

Drug therapy may be initiated to control the diarrhea, thereby reducing the risk of complications. Locally or systemically acting drugs may be recommended or prescribed. A list of commonly used locally acting substances follows. Two additional drugs, diphenoxylate with atropine and loperamide, are discussed in detail.

Locally acting antidiarrheal drugs

Drug	Dosage	Specific action
Aluminum hydroxide gel	30 ml	Adsorbent
Bismuth subsalicylate	60 to 120 mg	Adsorbent-protective
Kaolin mixture with pectin	30 ml	Adsorbent-hydrophilic
Psyllium hydrophilic mucilloid	4 to 10 gm	Hydrophilic-adsorbent
Polycarbophil	1 to 1.5 gm	Hydrophilic-adsorbent

Systemically active drugs may be prescribed, such as the opiate, paregoric, or the antiperistaltic meperidine derivatives, diphenoxylate and loperamide.

Systemically acting antidiarrheal drugs
Diphenoxylate and atropine

Drug action. Diphenoxylate inhibits gastrointestinal motility through its antiperistaltic effect; atropine has an antimuscarinic activity that discourages abuse.

Drug	Dosage
Diphenoxylate and atropine tablets	Initial: one to two tablets (2.5 to 5 mg of diphenoxylate) three to four times daily. Maintenance: one tablet (2.5 mg of diphenoxylate) two to three times daily as needed.

Proper use and precautions
1. Medication must be taken exactly as directed.
2. Decreased doses are recommended for the elderly and persons with impaired hepatic function or respiratory function.
3. Drug may be taken with food if it causes gastric distress.
4. Because of the dangers of accidental overdose in children, the drug must be kept out of their reach.
5. If diarrhea does not stop or a fever occurs, the physician should be notified.
6. Tolerance or dependence may develop with prolonged use.
7. Before any type of surgery, the physician or dentist should be informed about the drug.
8. Because the medication may cause dizziness or drowsiness, the patient should be cautioned about driving or operating mechanical household appliances.
9. Because of adverse effects, the patient should be cautioned against the use of alcohol, over-the-counter drugs, and other prescribed drugs.

10. Reduction of gastric motility in persons with travelers' diarrhea may result in fever caused by slow expulsion of infectious organisms that penetrate intestinal mucosa.
11. The medication should be used with caution for persons with many health problems.
12. Following prolonged administration, the drug should be withdrawn slowly to prevent withdrawal symptoms.
13. Drug interactions that may occur include alcohol, general anesthetics, other CNS depressants, tricyclic antidepressants (may increase CNS depression), haloperidol, phenothiazines, procainamide, quinidine (may increase effects of atropine), and antimuscarinics (may increase effects of diphenoxylate or atropine, producing paralytic ileus).
14. Side effects that may occur include symptoms of overdosage: loss of consciousness, shallow breathing, unusual excitement, and pinpoint pupils. Other effects requiring medical attention are loss of appetite, bloating, constipation, nausea, vomiting, and stomach pain. Other side effects are blurred vision, dry skin and mouth, fever, flushing, rapid heartbeat, restlessness, decreased urination, dizziness, drowsiness, depression, headache, numb hands or feet, skin rash, and swollen gums.
15. Monitoring consists of regular physician visits in long-term therapy.

Loperamide

Drug action. Loperamide inhibits peristaltic activity by a direct effect on muscles of the intestinal wall and also slows gastric motility.

Drug	Dosage
Loperamide	Acute diarrhea: initially 4 mg followed by 2 mg after each unformed stool until diarrhea is controlled.
	Chronic diarrhea: initially 4 mg followed by 2 mg after each unformed stool until diarrhea is controlled.
	Maintenance: 4 to 8 mg daily in single or divided doses.
	Maximum dose: 16 mg daily.

Proper use and precautions
1. Medication is to be taken exactly as directed.
2. Smaller doses are recommended for older persons with impaired hepatic function.
3. Neither tolerance nor dependence has been reported in humans.
4. If diarrhea does not stop or fever occurs, the physician should be notified.

5. In acute diarrhea, treatment with this drug should be discontinued if there is no improvement after 48 hours. In chronic diarrhea, if no improvement is noted after 10 days of therapy with the maximum dose, this drug is probably not effective.
6. Reduction of gastric motility in persons with travelers' diarrhea may result in fever caused by slow expulsion of infectious organisms that penetrate intestinal mucosa.
7. No drug interactions have been reported.
8. Side effects that may occur include dizziness, dry mouth, lack of appetite, nausea and vomiting, constipation, stomach pain, fever, drowsiness, and skin rash.
9. Monitoring consists of regular physician visits in long-term therapy.

REFERENCES

Bartal, M., and Heitkemper, M.: Gastrointestinal problems. In Carnavali, D., and Patrick, M., editors: Nursing management for the elderly, Philadelphia, 1975, J.B. Lippincott Co.
Lamy, P.: Prescribing for the elderly, Littleton, Mass., 1979, PSG Publishing Co., Inc.
Wuest, R., and Gossel, T.: Antacids, U.S. Pharmacist **6:**18, 1981.

SUGGESTED READINGS

Conrad, K.A., and Bressler, R., editors: Drug therapy for the elderly, St. Louis, 1981, The C.V. Mosby Co.
Strauss, B.: Disorders of the digestive system. In Rossman, I., editor: Clinical geriatrics, Philadelphia, 1979, J.B. Lippincott Co.

14

MANAGEMENT OF SELECTED URINARY PROBLEMS

Illnesses affecting the urinary system have an impact on the daily living patterns of older adults. The chronicity of incontinence and urinary tract infections greatly affects the total health picture for elderly persons. The health problems included in this section are urinary tract infections and incontinence.

URINARY TRACT INFECTIONS

The incidence of urinary tract infections increases in older persons. Brocklehurst (1979) found that urinary infections were present in about 20% of all women over 65 and that the incidence in men increased sharply 5 to 10 years later. In addition to age, a variety of other factors make older persons vulnerable to urinary infections. The presence of residual urine in the bladder because of an obstruction within the genitourinary system dilutes the normal urinary acidity, reducing its bacteriostatic effects, and an infection results. Diabetic patients prone to many infections and persons with renal failure are also susceptible. Persons with indwelling catheters, particularly if principles of asepsis are not practiced and if there is not a closed urinary drainage system, are prime candidates for infections. Institutionalized patients show a higher incidence than community-based populations, which may relate to any of the previously mentioned risk factors. Cross-contamination may also occur more readily in this debilitated group.

Signs and symptoms

Vague, nonspecific symptoms may confuse the practitioner in attempting to diagnose a urinary tract infection. It is possible that the person is asymptomatic. However, many old persons experience the classic symptoms of urinary frequency with urgency, dysuria, lower abdominal discomfort, and cloudy urine. Chills and fever, vomiting, hematuria, and urinary retention may also be present. Urine cultures should be done to isolate the bacteria, confirm the diagnosis, and define the therapy.

Management

Because of the high incidence of urinary tract infections in older persons, the practitioner should be alert to any of the signs and symptoms, such as change in voiding patterns, that could indicate an infection. In the event of an infection, fluids should be increased to 2500 to 3000 ml to ensure a urinary output of 1500 ml. Whether the patient is at home or in an institution, this plan can be instituted unless the cardiac status limits fluid intake. Regular voiding patterns should be promoted. The person should be instructed to lean forward when voiding, which will decrease the amount of urine that remains in the bladder. If incontinence does occur, the patient's perineal area should be carefully washed and dried. Because the soiled clothing and linen may harbor bacteria, these materials should be carefully handled to prevent contamination of other articles or persons who may live in the same environment.

The sulfonamides are frequently used in treating bacteriuria because of the high incidence of gram-negative urinary infections. Antimicrobial therapy is generally short term. In long-term therapy in which the goal is to prevent or reduce the frequency of the attacks, methenamine salts and nitrofurantoin are generally prescribed.

Drug therapy for urinary tract infections
Methenamine

Drug action. In an acid urine, methenamine is hydrolyzed to ammonia and formaldehyde, which is bactericidal.

Drug	Dosage
Methenamine tablets	1 gm q.6h.
Methenamine hippurate tablets	1 gm q.12h.

Proper use and precautions
1. Medication may be taken after meals and at bedtime if it causes nausea or an upset stomach.
2. A full course of treatment is necessary to achieve therapeutic effectiveness.
3. Urine should be checked daily and be maintained at an acid level with pH of 5 or below. Patients should be instructed how to perform this simple procedure.

4. To help maintain an acid urine the following foods should be increased: cranberries, plums, prunes, meat, fish, and eggs. Cranberry juice with supplemental vitamin C is recommended. To help prevent the formation of alkaline urine the following foods should be avoided: milk, nuts, fruits (including citrus fruits), vegetables, and antacids.
5. If symptoms do not improve within a few days, the patient should be instructed to contact the physician.
6. Drug interactions that may occur include alkalizing agents, antacids, carbonic anhydrase inhibitors, thiazide diuretics (may cause alkaline urine, rendering methenamine ineffective), and sulfonamides (concurrent use may result in crystalluria).
7. Side effects may include hematuria, dysuria, low back pain, rash, and gastric upset.
8. Monitoring includes daily testing of urine to determine acidity and adequacy of fluid intake.

Nitrofurantoin

Drug action. Nitrofurantoin is bacteriostatic in low concentrations and bactericidal in higher concentrations.

Drug	Dosage
Nitrofurantoin	Therapeutic: 50 to 100 mg q.6h.
	Prophylactic: 50 to 100 mg at bedtime

Proper use and precautions
1. Medication should be taken with food or milk to lessen gastric irritation and increase absorption.
2. Patient should be instructed to void before taking the bedtime dose, which will allow urine that is formed during the night to have a higher concentration of the drug.
3. A full course of treatment is necessary to achieve therapeutic effectiveness.
4. The drug may cause the urine to become rust-yellow to brown.
5. The medication may cause false-positive reactions in urine glucose testing.
6. If an oral liquid form of the medication is taken, the mouth should be rinsed immediately following administration to prevent staining of the teeth.
7. Drug interactions that may occur include nalidixic acid (may antagonize effects of nitrofurantoin) and probenecid (may inhibit renal tubular secretion of nitrofurantoin, resulting in increased serum levels and decreased urinary levels).
8. Side effects that may occur include chest pains, chills, fever, cough,

dizziness, drowsiness, headache, weakness, facial or oral burning, numbness, or tingling, pale or yellow skin, anorexia, nausea, vomiting, and diarrhea.
9. Monitoring includes regular physician visits, initial renal function tests, and signs of peripheral neuropathy if therapy is prolonged.

Sulfamethoxazole and trimethoprim

Drug action. Trimethoprim helps to create a lack of metabolically active folate, which increases the activity of sulfamethoxazole and expands its antibacterial spectrum.

Drug	Dosage
Sulfamethoxazole and trimethoprim	
Tablets	800 mg sulfamethoxazole and
Oral suspension	160 mg trimethoprim q.12h.

Proper use and precautions
1. Medication should be taken with a full glass of water 1 hour before meals or 2 hours after meals.
2. Fluid intake should be increased to a level that will provide 1200 to 1500 ml urinary output.
3. A full course of treatment is necessary to achieve maximum effectiveness.
4. An overgrowth of nonsusceptible organisms may occur.
5. Exposure to sun or a sunlamp should be avoided, because sensitivity to sun may occur while taking this medication and for months afterwards.
6. Before any type of surgery, the physician or dentist should be notified about the medication.
7. Drug interactions that may occur include urine-alkalinizing agents (increase solubility of sulfonamide), aminobenzoic acid (antagonizes bacteriostatic effect of sulfonamides), oral anticoagulants, oral hypoglycemic agents, methotrexate, phenytoin, thiopental (sulfonamides heighten or prolong effects of other drugs, increasing danger of toxicity), methenamine (increases danger of crystalluria), and probenecid (may decrease tubular secretion of sulfonamides, resulting in increased serum levels).
8. Side effects that may occur include photosensitivity, headache, rash, aching joints and muscles, difficulty in swallowing, fever, sore throat, redness, blistering, peeling or loosening of skin, yellowing of skin or eyes, fatigue or weakness, hematuria, dysuria, low back pain, swelling in anterior neck, anorexia, nausea, vomiting, and diarrhea.
9. Monitoring includes complete blood counts on a monthly basis and urinalysis on a regular basis.

INCONTINENCE

The problem of incontinence in older persons can remove them from the mainstream of life to self-imposed isolation. The involuntary escape of urine from the lower urinary tract is usually caused by an underlying factor, which properly treated or managed can have a positive influence on the person's life.

The prevalence varies, with institutionalized patients having a higher incidence than persons living at home. Few studies indicate the percentage of well elderly with incontinence, but Shanas (1979) and Wells (1980) in their studies reported that 50% to 55% of the older institutionalized population is incontinent. In addition, this group is vulnerable because of pathological changes such as urinary infections, enlarged prostate, cystocele, and vaginitis.

The risk factors offer clues to the causes of incontinence in older persons. The causes may be categorized into four groups: physical, emotional, environmental, and drugs. The physical changes are primarily associated with the genitourinary tract and include urinary tract infections, decreased muscle tone, obstruction caused by an enlarged prostate gland, vaginitis, urethritis, and fecal impaction. Emotional factors contributing to the development of incontinence include isolation, depression, sensory deprivation, regression, and attention seeking. The environmental factors are responsible for delays in reaching toilet facilities. Examples include long distance to the bathroom, inability to locate a bathroom, lack of safety aids in toilet, and unsuitable clothing and footwear. Drugs that may affect incontinence include diuretics, hypnotics, sedatives, antianxiety agents, and antidepressants.

Signs and symptoms

Because of the stigma attached to incontinence, the subject is not discussed, and the evidence is frequently concealed. However, the odor of urine, soiled clothing, or reluctance to participate in social activities may indicate this problem.

Management

The first step in the management of incontinence is to refer the person to an appropriate practitioner for diagnosis of the cause of the problem, followed by the development of a plan for management. Health practitioners may be involved with patients who have this sensitive problem, and the following suggestions are offered (Brink, 1980). Further reading is recommended.

- Approximately 2500 ml of fluids should be taken daily unless contraindicated by another medical problem.

- Fluids should be discontinued after 8 PM, except when the weather is hot or the person is active.
- Caffeine-containing fluids such as coffee, tea, and cola should be eliminated because of their diuretic effects.
- The bladder should be emptied at regularly scheduled intervals throughout the day and also when the person feels the need to void.
- Diuretics should be taken early in the morning.
- Exercises to strengthen the pelvic muscles and sphincters should be done on a regular, prescribed schedule.
- Sanitary pads and protective briefs or pants should be used. The skin should be washed with mild soap and water on a regular basis.
- A regular bowel program should be established. Intake of high-fiber foods should be encouraged.

Drug therapy is effective in managing incontinence. A physician skilled in diagnosing the type of incontinence should be consulted to define the appropriate drug therapy. Finkbeiner (1980) suggests that drugs used to treat incontinence include cholinergics to increase bladder emptying, anticholinergics to decrease bladder hyperactivity related to neurological causes, antispasmodics to decrease bladder irritation, α-adrenergics to increase outlet resistance, and α-adrenergic blocking agents to decrease outlet resistance. More commonly used drugs described in this section include bethanechol, propantheline, methantheline, oxybutyrin, and phenylpropanolamine.

Drugs used in incontinence
Cholinergic agent: bethanechol

Drug action. Bethanechol mimics acetylcholine and stimulates cholinergic receptors; it promotes bladder emptying by increasing intravesical pressure or eliciting contraction.

Drug	Dosage
Bethanechol	Oral: 50 to 100 mg q.i.d. Subcutaneous: 2.5 to 10 mg q.2½h.

Proper use and precautions
1. Sterile solution is for subcutaneous route only. Administration by other parenteral routes may produce violent cholinergic overstimulation.
2. Maximum effect of the oral route occurs in 1 hour and disappears in 2 to 6 hours.
3. Oral doses exceeding 100 mg every 4 to 6 hours may cause additive effects.
4. Medication is contraindicated or used with caution for persons with an

anatomical obstruction of the bladder outlet, hyperthyroidism, peptic ulcer, asthma, coronary artery disease, epilepsy, parkinsonism, and pronounced bradycardia and hypotension.

5. Drug interactions that may occur include ganglionic blocking compounds (may cause a critical drop in blood pressure).
6. Side effects that may occur include lacrimation, salivation, sweating, flushing, abdominal cramps, diarrhea, nausea, belching, headache, and difficulty in visual accommodation.
7. Monitoring of desirable and undesirable effects is recommended during the first 48 hours of therapy.

Anticholinergic agents: propantheline and methantheline

Drug action. Propantheline and methantheline compete with acetylcholine for cholinergic receptors and decrease bladder activity; they are used for incontinence caused by neurological impairment.

Drug	Dosage
Propantheline	Oral: 15 to 30 mg t.i.d. or q.i.d.
Methantheline	Oral: 50 to 100 mg t.i.d. or q.i.d.

Proper use and precautions. Refer to Chapter 13.

Antispasmodic agent: oxybutynin

Drug action. Oxybutynin directly depresses bladder smooth muscle, producing a local anesthesia; it is useful for urge incontinence caused by bladder irritation.

Drug	Dosage
Oxybutynin	5 mg t.i.d. or q.i.d.

Proper use and precautions
1. Oxybutynin is used with caution for the elderly and persons with impaired renal or hepatic function.
2. Medication should not be administered in high environmental temperature because of the danger of heat prostration.
3. Because drowsiness and blurred vision may occur, patients should be cautioned about driving a car and operating mechanical equipment.
4. Symptoms of hyperthyroidism, coronary artery disease and other cardiac problems, hypertension, and prostatic hypertrophy may be aggravated by this medication.
5. Side effects may include dry mouth, decreased sweating, blurred vision, mydriasis, constipation, restlessness, insomnia, nausea, vomiting, bloating, allergenic reactions, and urticaria.

α-Adrenergic agent: phenylpropanolamine

Drug action. Phenylpropanolamine stimulates α-adrenergic receptors of bladder outlet and increases bladder outlet resistance; it is used in stress incontinence.

Drug	Dosage
Phenylpropanolamine capsule	25 to 50 mg t.i.d. or q.i.d.
Phenylpropanolamine timed-release capsule	One capsule b.i.d.

Proper use and precautions
1. Risk of dizziness, drowsiness, and hypotension is greater in persons over 60 years of age.
2. Because drowsiness may occur, patients should be cautioned about driving a car or operating mechanical equipment.
3. Alcohol should be avoided, because CNS depression may occur.
4. Drug interactions that may occur include alcohol, other CNS depressants (increase CNS depression), and MAO inhibitors (produce marked hypertension).
5. Side effects that may occur include dry mouth, rash, weakness, angina, hypertension or hypotension, tightness in chest, drowsiness, nervousness, insomnia, irritability, incoordination, gastric distress, nausea, vomiting, and difficulty in urination.

REFERENCES

Brink, C.: Assessing the problem, Geriatr. Nurs. **1:**241, 1980.
Brocklehurst, J.: The urinary tract. In Rossman, I., editor: Clinical geriatrics, ed. 2, Philadelphia, 1979, J.B. Lippincott Co.
Finkbeiner, A.: Helpful drugs, Geriatr. Nurs. **1:**270, 1980.
Shanas, E.: The family as a support system, Gerontologist **19:**170, 1979.
Wells, T.: Problems in geriatric nursing care, Edinburgh, 1980, Churchill Livingstone.

SUGGESTED READINGS

Cotterel, M., and Miller, M.: Nursing implications of drug therapy, Geriatr. Nurs. **1:**271, 1980.
Demmerle, B., and Bartol, A.: Nursing care of the incontinent patient, Geriatr. Nurs. **1:**246, 1980.
Dufault, S.: Urinary incontinence: United States and British nursing perspectives, J. Gerontol. Nurs. **4:**28, March/April 1978.
Mandelstam, D., and others: Special techniques, Geriatr. Nurs. **1:**251, 1980.
Willington, F.: Urinary incontinence: a practical approach, Geriatrics **35:**41, 1980.

MANAGEMENT OF SELECTED
EYE PROBLEMS

15

Visual changes become more pronounced as persons grow older, but 80% to 85% of elderly adults have good to adequate visual acuity up to the age of 90 (Kornzweig, 1979). However, with advancing age, persons become more vulnerable to certain pathological conditions such as cataracts, glaucoma, and macular degeneration. This chapter will explore the etiological factors associated with eye changes, aspects of prevention, and visual changes known to be responsive to drug therapy—wide-angle glaucoma, narrow-angle glaucoma, and dry eyes. The therapeutic treatment by medication for each of these problems will be discussed.

The ocular side effects of medications to which older adults are particularly vulnerable have been presented throughout these sections concerning drug therapy. These systemic drugs that are frequently given on a chronic basis may not be dose adjusted for the older person, and as a result, eye changes occur. Drugs that are especially problematic include antidepressants, cardiovascular drugs, anticholinergics, and the phenothiazines. Chronic illnesses of older persons are frequently controlled by these medications; therefore the practitioner must be aware of the visual side effects to advise the patient as well as other practitioners who may be providing care.

Health practitioners also have an opportunity to refer older persons to qualified ophthalmologists, who are knowledgeable about the eye changes in the elderly, for regular programs of eye care. Advising clients to use free glaucoma screening programs sponsored by the National Society for the Prevention of Blindness will also help reduce the incidence of blindness caused by glaucoma.

GLAUCOMA

The second most significant eye problem in aging persons is glaucoma, which shows a significant increase between the ages of 40 and 65 years. The

National Society for the Prevention of Blindness (1977) reported that when 53,021 persons over 55 were screened, 5.3% were referred for further examination. Glaucoma was found in 405 persons and was suspected in 806 persons. This latter group was considered borderline and likely to develop glaucoma. Because of the incidence of this eye defect, all eye and physical examinations should include tonometry readings. Because glaucoma has a hereditary tendency, persons with a family history should have an annual examination. The two types of glaucoma, wide-angle and narrow-angle, vary in onset, signs and symptoms, and treatment. Common to both types of glaucoma is an abnormally high intraocular pressure that can lead to progressive loss of vision resulting from damage to the optic nerve. Treatment is directed at decreasing intraocular pressure.

WIDE-ANGLE GLAUCOMA

Wide-angle glaucoma, the most common type, develops slowly and insidiously over a period of years, is not painful, and is frequently discovered after visual changes have occurred. This type of glaucoma occurs as a result of changes in the area of Schlemm's canal. The fluid backs up, causing a painless increase in intraocular pressure, which affects the retina and optic nerve. Without treatment these changes lead to a progressive loss of the visual field.

Signs and symptoms

Wide-angle glaucoma is usually discovered on a routine examination and has vague symptoms that may include change in visual acuity, feeling of eyestrain, and morning headache that disappears. On examination the signs include elevated intraocular pressure, change in the angle formed by the cornea and iris, visual field defect, and damage to the optic nerve. Therapy is directed at reducing the elevated intraocular pressure by decreasing the production of fluid or increasing the outflow of fluid.

NARROW-ANGLE GLAUCOMA

Narrow-angle glaucoma occurs in the fifth and sixth decades of life and is more common in women. It is thought that persons with a shallow anterior chamber are anatomically predisposed to this type of glaucoma. As persons grow older, the lens continues to grow and increase in size. As a result, the chamber narrows. Persons with this shallow chamber are particularly vulnerable to the effects of anticholinergic and sympathomimetic drugs, with or without glaucoma.

Signs and symptoms

Narrow-angle glaucoma has an acute onset, and treatment is urgent to prevent blindness. High intraocular pressure is caused by a complete closure of the drain angle by the iris. Symptoms that may be reported by the patient include intense eye pain, nausea, blurred vision, and red and green halos around lights. Signs visible to the practitioner include injected, watery looking eyes and dilated pupils.

Immediate treatment is directed at constricting the iris with the use of miotic drops. The use of carbonic anhydrase inhibitors or hyperosmolar solutions will cause diuresis and as a result will slow the production of aqueous fluid. Surgery may be necessary if the pressure cannot be relieved.

MANAGEMENT

The goal of therapy for glaucoma is to maintain the intraocular pressure within normal limits either by decreasing the rate of production of fluid or increasing the rate of outflow. The primary therapy is the use of miotic drops that aid in outflow by constricting the pupil and widening the drain angle.

Various types of miotics, short-acting parasympathomimetics, and short-acting and long-acting anticholinesterase compounds are generally prescribed. However, in some circumstances the intraocular pressure cannot be controlled completely with miotics, and adrenergic drugs may be used. Medications such as epinephrine and phenylephrine produce an additive drop in pressure by vasoconstriction of the ocular vessels. The use of a β-adrenergic antagonist is also effective in producing greater reduction of intraocular pressure with fewer local or systemic side effects.

During acute attacks of glaucoma the pressure may continue to rise but is responsive to carbonic anhydrase inhibitors such as acetazolamide, which may be used in conjunction with miotics and adrenergic vasoconstrictors. In situations in which the pressure does not respond to this therapy, osmotic diuretic agents (mannitol and urea) may be indicated. These drugs act by increasing the osmotic pressure of the blood plasma to a level above the aqueous humor and vitreous body. Fluid from the eye then flows into the hyperosmotic plasma and reduces the intraocular pressure.

Topical drugs
Miotics

Drug action. Miotics act by directly or indirectly causing the muscles of the iris and ciliary body to contract, which pulls the structures away from the angle opening up the meshwork of small channels that drain into Schlemm's canal. Constriction of the pupil thins the iris, pulling it out of the angle.

Drugs	Dosage
Short-acting parasympathomimetics	
Carbachol	1 gtt of 0.75% to 3% solution, one to four times daily.
Pilocarpine nitrate	1 gtt of 0.5% to 6% solution, one to six times daily.

Drugs	Dosage
Short-acting anticholinesterase compounds	
Neostigmine bromide	1 to 2 gtts of 0.25% to 5% solution, two to six times daily.
Physostigmine sulfate	1 gtt of 0.25% to 1% solution, up to four times daily.

Drugs	Dosage
Long-acting anticholinesterase compounds*	
Demecarium bromide	1 to 2 gtts of 0.25% solution, one to two times daily (or less).
Echothiophate iodide	1 gtt of 0.06% to 0.25% solution, one to two times daily.

Adrenergic agents

Drug action. In some circumstances intraocular pressure cannot be completely controlled with miotics, and adrenergic agents may be used. Instillation of this type of drug after the use of a miotic produces an additive drop in the pressure by its effect on the ocular vessels.

Drugs	Dosage
Epinephrine	1 gtt of 0.5% to 2% solution every 12 to 24 hours.
Phenylephrine	1 gtt of 0.125% to 10% solution, every 12 to 24 hours.

Adrenergic blocking agents

Drug action. Adrenergic blocking agents reduce formation of aqueous humor and increase outflow of humor.

Drug	Dosage
Timolol maleate	1 gtt of 0.25% to 0.5% solution two times daily

*Generally not administered in narrow-angle glaucoma, because these drugs produce a powerful, contracting action on the sphincter and iris that may cause congestion by pushing these muscles against other ocular structures. This action may decrease the flow from the congested angle.

Side effects of topical drugs used in glaucoma*

 I. Cholinergic miotics
   A. Ocular effects—early
     1. Stinging sensation
     2. Tearing
     3. Eyelid twitching
     4. Dimming of vision in poor light
     5. Blurring of vision
     6. Headache
     7. Possible pupillary block caused by paradoxical ocular hypertension
   B. Ocular effects—late
     1. Conjunctivitis
     2. Conjunctival thickening
     3. Nasolacrimal duct and canal obstruction
     4. Lens opacities
   C. Systemic effects
     1. Nausea, vomiting, abdominal cramps, diarrhea
     2. Bronchoconstriction, wheezing, chest tightness
     3. Bradycardia and hypotension
     4. Salivation, sweating
 II. Adrenergic agents
   A. Ocular effects
     1. Stinging, tearing
     2. Occasional initial blanching followed by hyperemia
     3. Pigmented deposits
     4. Angle closure in persons with narrow-angle glaucoma
   B. Systemic effects
     1. Tachycardia, palpitations
     2. Hypertension (especially in persons taking MAO inhibitors and tricyclic antidepressants)
III. Adrenergic blocking agents
   A. Ocular effects
     1. Mild irritation
   B. Systemic effects
     1. Decrease in resting heart rate
     2. Used with caution in persons with cardiac problems and bronchial asthma

Systemic drugs

Carbonic anhydrase inhibitors

Drug action. Carbonic anhydrase inhibitors inhibit action of the enzyme cabonic anhydrase, which affects ocular fluid formation.

Drug	Dosage
Acetazolamide	Oral: 250 mg, two to four times daily. Parenteral: 500 mg followed by 250 mg every 4 hours.

*Adapted from Rodman, M., and Smith, D.: Pharmacology and drug therapy, ed. 3, Philadelphia, 1979, J.B. Lippincott Co.

Side effects of systemic drugs used in glaucoma

Anorexia, nausea and vomiting, abdominal discomfort
Headache, drowsiness, confusion
Paresthesias of the hands or feet or around the mouth
Frequent urination, hypokalemia, hyperuricemia
Renal calculus
Skin rashes, fever, bone marrow depression

• • •

When counseling the older person with glaucoma, the practitioner should stress that glaucoma treatment must be continued for the remainder of life, because the defect is not cured but is controlled with eye drops. The drops must be instilled at regular intervals. To facilitate the regularity, using some routine activities as a reminder has proven to be a successful mechanism. Explaining that the pressure rises as the pupil dilates and that the pupil dilates while asleep will help the person understand that drops must be instilled at bedtime, on arising, and at additional intervals as prescribed. The constricted pupils will also decrease the ability to see in the dark, and night driving should be discouraged. The use of night lights is also recommended.

When eye drops or ointments are prescribed, the patient should be instructed regarding appropriate administration. Drops are carefully placed in a sac made by gently everting the lower lid, instead of placing the drops onto the sensitive cornea. The patient then gently closes his eyelids. When applying eye ointment the patient should look upward while placing a thin ribbon of ointment on the inner surface of the lower lid. The eyelids should be closed gently and massaged very lightly to spread the ointment. Whether administering drops or ointment, care must be exercised to avoid touching the equipment to the eye, which may cause injury as well as contamination of the container.

DRY EYES

The most common external eye disease, especially among older women, is dryness of the eyes because of impaired tearing. Previously considered a process limited to postmenopausal women, the condition can occur at any age in both sexes. The dryness is known to increase with age and is the source of a great deal of discomfort with older persons.

The patient may complain of a dry sensation, burning, smarting, scratching, and eye fatigue. The symptoms become more pronounced at the end of the day, especially if the air is dry or the person is in a draft. The conjunctiva may appear reddened and moist, and in more advanced cases it takes on a velvetlike redness with thickened mucous threads. Mild infections may accompany this condition, which exaggerates symptoms previously described.

The treatment of dry eyes is directed toward keeping the eyes moist and eliminating infections if present. Among the agents used to treat dry eye are those that increase tear viscosity (methylcellulose) and agents that produce a filmlike corneal covering (polyvinyl alcohol). A disadvantage of methylcellulose is the flaky residue that is left, which combines with mucus, decreasing vision and causing discomfort. Because of the short duration of action, the instillation of these agents, known as artificial tears, must take place frequently during the day. The use of a greasy ointment such as Lacri-lube instilled at bedtime relieves some of the symptoms by forming a thin film similar to the natural lipid layer of natural tears. The discomfort associated with this condition becomes discouraging, because therapy is limited to comfort measures.

REFERENCES

Kornzweig, A.: The eye in old age. In Rossman, I., editor: Clinical geriatrics, Philadelphia, 1979, J.B. Lippincott Co.

National Society for the Prevention of Blindness: Annual bulletin, 1977.

SUGGESTED READINGS

Boyer, G.: Vision problems. In Carnevali, D., and Patrick, M., editors: Nursing management for the elderly, Philadelphia, 1979, J.B. Lippincott Co.

Bucek, S.: Visual status of the elderly, J. Gerontol. Nurs. **2:**36, 1976.

Hatton, J.: Aging and the glare problem, J. Gerontol. Nurs. **3:**38, 1977.

Dangel, M., and Havener, W.: Drugs and the aging eye, Geriatrics **36:**133, 1981.

Rodman, M., and Smith, D.: Pharmacology and drug therapy in nursing, ed. 3, Philadelphia, 1979, J.B. Lippincott Co.

Yurick, A., and others: The aged person and the nursing process, New York, 1980, Appleton-Century-Crofts.

16

MANAGEMENT OF SELECTED SKIN PROBLEMS

Skin disorders continue to be a problem for older adults and are compounded by the changes that take place as part of the aging process. The incidence of skin disorders is affected by climate, occupation, extent of melanin in the skin, and general state of health. Certain factors known to influence the development and course of disorders include impaired peripheral vascular circulation, altered response of nerve endings to sensory stimulation, poor nutrition, extensive solar exposure, decreased immune response, and use of varied drugs.

Skin changes associated with aging have been discussed previously, but the effect of some of these alterations on the development of skin problems is included in this chapter. Also included are the common problems of dry skin and pruritis, infectious problems such as herpes zoster and onychomycosis, skin tumors, drug-induced skin eruptions, and foot problems.

PRURITIS

Pruritis, or itching, is a very common complaint of older persons and can be aggravated by temperature changes, perspiration, fatigue, emotional upsets, and contact with clothing. It can be systemically caused in diseases such as hyperthyroidism, gout, liver disease, and chronic renal disease. Pruritis frequently accompanies drug reactions.

The pruritis that occurs most commonly is caused by dry skin, and measures to relieve dry skin may also be effective in relieving the itching. If rehydration of the stratum corneum does not relieve this aggravating symptom, cool compresses or oatmeal baths may prove effective, especially if followed by lubricating lotions. Vigorous rubbing with a rough towel or similar material will intensify the itching by stimulating the sensory nerve endings. If pruritis interferes with sleep, low doses of antihistamines may be prescribed for bedtime use.

DRY SKIN

Dry skin is probably the most common problem of aging, especially among persons who have a history of it and chapping. The skin change occurs as a result of decreased secretion of sebum, the substance produced by sebaceous glands, which in turn reduces the availability of the protective lipid film that retards evaporation from the stratum corneum. Because the epidermis thins with aging, moisture escapes through the skin. The dryness is compounded by inadequate fluid intake, nutritional deficiencies, exposure to the sun's rays and low humidity, the use of harsh soaps, and frequent hot baths.

Dry skin is evident on various parts of the body and may be manifested in various ways. The dry, flaky, scaly areas may be present on the exposed body parts, face, neck, hands, and forearms, as well as the trunk and thighs. The lower legs, where circulation may be slightly impaired, may be smooth and shiny with fine pink, moist fissures. Itching generally accompanies the dryness and may result in irritations or scratch marks. Because dry skin is considered a symptom, an evaluation is done to rule out systemic diseases and also the possibility of scabies and lice.

The management of dry skin is focused on rehydration of the dermis. Bathing with tepid water and using superfatted soaps such as Basis help to restore a thin lipid film to the skin surface. Bath oils help hold the moisture in the skin, but using them in the tub is not recommended because of the danger of slipping and falling. It is safer and probably more effective to apply the oil directly to the skin following a bath or shower. The application of lotions or emollients several times daily will also keep the skin lubricated; vegetable oils are also effective and inexpensive. Additional health measures that will protect the skin include maintaining adequate humidity, avoiding the use of rough clothing and linens, bathing less frequently, and drying the skin carefully.

FUNGAL INFECTIONS OF THE NAIL

Onychomycosis, a fungal infection of the toenail, is frequently seen in older persons. The nail becomes hypertrophied, opaque, and scaly. A flaky substance forms under the nail, pushing the central portion upward and forcing the sides of the nail into the toe, similar to an ingrown toenail. If a culture is positive for fungus, antifungal agents, topical or oral preparations, are recommended. In addition to griseofulvin, which is described on the opposite page, nystatin in powder or cream form may be applied directly to the nail bed. Keeping the area clean and dry also promotes healing and prevents reinfection.

Griseofulvin

Drug action. Griseofulvin is deposited in living cells, which are converted to keratin when they die; the presence of griseofulvin in the keratin layer acts as a barrier to further fungal growth; new cells grow out, pushing off the fungal infected tissues that are shed or clipped.

Drug	Dosage
Griseofulvin, microsize	500 mg to 1 gm daily.
Griseofulvin, ultramicrosize	330 mg daily or b.i.d.

Proper use and precautions
1. Medication should be taken with or after meals to decrease gastric irritation. Taking the dose at noon may increase absorption. In some circumstances, high-fat meals may be recommended to increase absorption.
2. Completing a full course of treatment as prescribed is necessary.
3. Medication may increase sensitivity to sunlight, necessitating avoidance of or protection from the sun's rays.
4. Drinking alcohol when taking this medication may cause tachycardia and flushing.
5. The infected area must be kept clean and dry to prevent reinfection.
6. Drug interactions that may occur include alcohol, barbiturates (decrease effects of griseofulvin), and coumarin-type anticoagulants (anticoagulant effects may be decreased).
7. Side effects include skin rash; hives; itching; sore mouth or tongue; numbness, tingling, pain, or weakness of hands or feet; sore throat or fever; headache; and confusion.
8. Monitoring includes regular physician visits and hematopoietic, liver, and renal function determination.

HERPES ZOSTER

Herpes zoster, caused by the varicella-zoster virus, is common in older persons. In children the illness is manifested as varicella; the virus may lie dormant in the dorsal root ganglia and years later exacerbate as herpes zoster.

This skin disorder is manifested by papulovesicular eruptions that follow a unilateral dermatome distribution, generally involving one arm or around one side of the lower chest. The pain, which may precede the eruption, and occurs with the eruption, is a burning type and often very severe. Depending on the location and severity, this condition can be quite incapacitating.

The disorder is usually self-limited and disappears in 3 to 4 weeks. Treatment is aimed at promoting comfort by relieving pain and caring for the lesions and depends on the severity of the illness. In a few cases pain, which can be severe, may persist after the eruption is over. Analgesics and psychiatric therapy may be necessary. In very severe conditions, a nerve block may be indicated.

BENIGN TUMORS OF THE SKIN

Four types of lesions are frequently referred to as the hallmark of old age, appearing after the age of 50. They are benign but frequently the source of questions from older persons who are concerned about malignant skin lesions.

Seborrheic keratoses

Seborrheic keratoses are common growths that appear primarily on the chest, back, face, and scalp. They are circumscribed, small, raised, flesh colored to darkly pigmented, and greasy looking. Because of the change in color, which is caused by melanin deposits, people fear that they may be malignant. They may be removed for cosmetic reasons.

Senile lentigines

Senile lentigines are small areas of pigmentation, commonly referred to as liver spots, that typically appear on sun-exposed areas of the face, hands, and forearms. No treatment is required, and the heavily advertised hormone creams have no effect on removing the discoloration.

Acrochordons

Acrochordons are small flesh-colored skin tags that occur around the neck, trunk, axilla, and groin. Treatment may be sought for cosmetic reasons or if clothing irritates the small skin tags.

Cherry angiomata

Cherry angiomata are tiny red lesions that commonly occur on the back and chest. They are small collections of capillaries and have no malignant potential.

MALIGNANT TUMORS OF THE SKIN

Squamous cell carcinoma and basal cell carcinoma are malignant tumors. The premalignant lesions of the skin, actinic or solar keratosis, occur commonly on sun-exposed parts of the body. The lesions appear as erythematous areas that are rough and scaly and on palpation may cause some discomfort. Because of the potential to become cancerous, early recognition and treatment are important.

Basal cell carcinoma

Basal cell carcinoma is most generally found on the face, but it also occurs on the trunk or extremities. It most frequently appears in fair-skinned persons in their sixties who have had much exposure to the sun. Several types of lesions may occur, but the most common is a raised nodular lesion that is waxy, shiny, and sometimes ulcerated. Early attention is necessary, but metastasis is rare.

Squamous cell carcinoma

Squamous cell carcinoma is more aggressive, with a higher incidence of metastasis. The nodule is flesh colored in the early stages and becomes reddened and scaly. It may be hard with a gray top of horny texture, or it may ulcerate. This carcinoma is most common in older, fair-skinned persons who have had sun exposure. Prompt treatment is necessary because of the danger of metastasis.

DRUG-INDUCED SKIN ERUPTIONS

Skin rashes are possible side effects of many of the drugs taken by older persons. The situation is complicated by the number and variety of medications that are administered to an individual in controlling chronic illnesses. When a rash occurs, the drug administered most recently is suspected. The type of eruption may also offer a clue when attempting to identify which drug is causing the reaction. Fisher (1979) identified the types of eruptions that are associated with 48 different drugs that are frequently taken by older persons. The eruptions generally occur within 1 week after the sensitizing drug is taken, except those that are caused by ampicillin and other semi-synthetic penicillins, which appear after 10 to 14 days.

When the practitioner or patient is aware of a skin eruption that may be drug related, the physician should be notified and the eruption described.

Discussing with the patient any drugs that may have been added to the regimen, either prescribed by a physician or purchased over the counter, will be helpful in isolating the offending drug. Fisher (1979) suggests the following general principles of care in treating cutaneous skin reactions.

- If possible, the suspected drug should be discontinued. If the drug is essential, another chemically unrelated drug with similar action should be substituted.
- Warm baths and the application of colloidal oatmeal are helpful for vesicular or oozing eruptions.
- Adding oil to the bath water is comforting for dry lesions.
- Low-dose antihistamines may be prescribed for the pruritis that may occur with the eruption.
- Systemic corticosteroids may be necessary in treating severe eruptions.

The patient who is informed of the possibility of skin eruptions caused by specific drugs is also the person who can seek treatment before the reaction becomes serious. The treatment will vary according to the stage and nature of the eruption and the presence of any systemic manifestations.

FOOT PROBLEMS

Foot problems in older persons can be the source of discomfort, fatigue, irritability, and chronic complaints. Schanck (1977) and Conrad (1977) found that in a community population, corns, calluses, toenail problems, bunions, edema, and fungus infections occurred most frequently.

Corns and calluses

Corns and calluses that occur on older persons' feet are similar to those occurring at any age. They occur as a protective response, since thicker skin can withstand more pressure and friction. Corns occurring over a bony prominence lead to a core that is directed inward and causes pain. Calluses form over the flat surfaces of the feet, especially the plantar surface, which increases pressure on the sole.

Older people have probably used the same method of removing corns and calluses for years, ranging from over-the-counter preparations to cutting them with a razor blade. These methods of treatment should be reassessed, because the treatment can be more disastrous than the original problem. Corn pads, a common remedy, actually increase the pressure on the area surrounding the corn, which can impair circulation and lead to tissue breakdown.

Foot care

The suggestions that follow will be helpful to practitioners who are often asked for advice about how to handle foot problems:

1. Inspect feet daily in good light. Use a mirror to view parts of the feet if necessary.
2. Wash feet daily with warm water and mild soap. Dry carefully, using a patting motion.
3. Lightly massage reddened areas with lanolin-type cream. If feet are dry and scaly, massage lightly with lanolin-type lotion. Avoid excess accumulation of lotions or creams on the feet.
4. Avoid use of strong medication to remove corns and calluses. After soaking feet, calluses may be rubbed with a fine emery board or piece of sandpaper. Pressure should be relieved from corns and calluses by adjustments to shoes.
5. If toenails are hard, making them difficult to cut, soak feet in water before caring for them. Use toenail clippers, cutting straight across the nail.
6. Avoid wearing clothing or shoes that may restrict circulation.
7. Avoid exposing feet to extreme temperatures such as hot water bottles or heating pads. Check the bath water temperature with your hand before getting into the tub.
8. If visual deficits or immobility prevent proper self-foot care, a family member should be instructed about how to provide the service.
9. Consult a podiatrist or physician for problems that may be encountered.
10. These guidelines may need to be adapted for diabetic patients and people with circulatory problems.

REFERENCES

Conrad, D.: Foot education and screening programs for the elderly, J. Gerontol. Nurs. **3**:11, 1977.
Fisher, A.: Drug-induced skin eruptions: typical treatments for topical problems, Geriatrics **34**: 79, 1979.
Schanck, M.: A survey of the well-elderly: their foot problems, practices, and needs, J. Gerontol. Nurs. **3**:10, 1977.

SUGGESTED READINGS

Carnevali, D., and Patrick, M.: Nursing management for the elderly, Philadelphia, 1979, J.B. Lippincott Co.
Crupps, D.: Skin care and problems in the aged, Hosp. Pract. **12**:119, 1977.
Hanifin, J.: Eczematous conditions in the elderly: common and curable, Geriatrics **34**:29, 1979.

EPILOGUE

Health professionals educated today will be increasingly more involved in the health care of the older population. As people live to an older age and patterns of health care change, practitioners will have an increasing need to be prepared to work with older adults. Academic programs have a responsibility to provide broad-based programs in gerontology that include an opportunity to develop skills required for working with older persons.

Changes in the health-care system will provide new sites for practitioners to use their expertise. They can expect to function in new roles in retirement communities, multiservice senior centers, nutrition sites, day-care centers, day hospitals, and the more traditional settings of community pharmacies, nursing homes, and hospitals. Health maintenance and restoration will continue to be the focus of health care, but a new emphasis will be placed on prevention.

Members of each health discipline will encounter problems and concerns that older adults have about coping with often complicated medication regimens. In some situations, immediate problem solving may be feasible. Other circumstances will require referral to the person who has the most expertise about the subject. Interdisciplinary communication will become increasingly essential.

Having a broad knowledge base in the field of gerontology, demonstrating interest in working directly with older adults, assuming new roles in the health-care system, and possessing the expertise in interdisciplinary planning provide the challenges for the future as we encounter growing numbers of older people.

INDEX

Cushing's syndrome and secondary osteoporosis, 135
Cyclic AMP; *see* Adenosine monophosphate
Cyclic GMP; *see* Guanosine monophosphate, 180
Cyclophosphamide and allopurinol, 51
Cycloserine and vitamin B$_6$ deficiency, 76
Cystocele and incontinence, 207
Cytoxan; *see* Cyclophosphamide
Cytotoxic drugs, 77

D

Dalmane; *see* Flurazepam
Danthron, dosage of, 197
Darvon; *see* Propoxyphene
Death, leading causes of, in older adults, 3
Decisions, encouraging older persons to participate in, 91
Deficiencies, drug-induced nutrient, in older persons, 75-77
Dehydration, 74
  and arrhythmias, 159
  and reduction in renal blood flow and glomerular filtration rate, 29
Delirium, 49
Demecarium bromide, dosage of, 214
Demerol; *see* Meperidine
Demographics of gerontology, 1-4
Dental hygiene, poor, as cause of tooth loss, 17
Dentures, ill-fitting, affecting digestion, 17
Depen; *see* Penicillamine
Dependency
  and benzodiazepines, 107
  on laxatives, 198
Depot injections, 27
Depression, 45
  and anxiety, 106
  bipolar, 101
  causes of, 101-102
  chemicals important in, 102
  clinical, 101
  endogenous, 101
  exogenous, 101
  and incontinence, 207
  management of, 103-106
  physiological signs in, 102
  psychological symptoms of, 102
  signs and symptoms of, 102
  situational, 101
  types of, 101
  unipolar, 101
Dermatitis, seborrheic, as result of drug-induced vitamin deficiency, 76
Dermis, rehydration of, 220

Desipramine, 43, 66
  for depression, 102
  dosage of, 104
Desyrel; *see* Trazodone
Detoxification, 24
Dexamethasone suppression test as diagnosis of depression, 102
Dextrothyroxine and sulfonylureas, 47
Diabetes and Aging, 141
Diabetes, 31
  as factor in atherosclerosis, 152
  fear of, in older adults, 54
  mellitus, 137-145
  prevalence of, among older adults, 3
  type I, 141
  type II, 141
Diabetic patients
  and nail and foot problems, 10
  and urinary tract infections, 203
  and vulnerability to tuberculosis, 186
Diabinese; *see* Chlorpropamide
Diagnosis
  incorrect, as problem of self-treatment, 55
  increased problems of, in older adults, 3
  making, 54
Diamox; *see* Acetazolamide
Diarrhea, 40
  drugs that may cause, 198-199
  and magnesium compounds, 193
  management of, 199-202
  medication-induced, 198
  signs and symptoms of, 199
Diazepam, 36
  decreased hepatic metabolism of, 28
  dosage of, 107
  elevated blood levels of, 37
Dicyclomine, 43
Diet
  and cardiovascular disease, 16
  in control of diabetes in older adult, 138-139
  low-calorie, 70
  in prevention of constipation, 197
Dietary allowances, recommended, for older persons, 80
Dietary history, 78
Digestion
  as factor affecting use of food in older adults, 75
  ill-fitting dentures affecting, 17
  lack of teeth affecting, 17
Digitalis glycosides and reduced renal function, 37
Digitalis therapy and arrhythmias, 159
Digitalis toxicity and excessive loss of potassium from diuretics, 38-39